Leaving the City

Health and Happiness in
the Other America

Leaving the City

Health and Happiness in the Other America

Jeffrey Tipton

EARTH
BOOKS

Winchester, UK
Washington, USA

JOHN HUNT PUBLISHING

First published by Earth Books, 2022
Earth Books is an imprint of John Hunt Publishing Ltd., No. 3 East St., Alresford,
Hampshire SO24 9EE, UK
office@jhpbooks.com
www.johnhuntpublishing.com
www.earth-books.net

For distributor details and how to order please visit the 'Ordering' section on our website.

Text copyright: Jeffrey Tipton 2021

ISBN: 978 1 78904 924 4
978 1 78904 925 1 (ebook)
Library of Congress Control Number: 2021947897

A CIP catalogue record for this book is available from the British Library.

Design: Matthew Greenfield

UK: Printed and bound by CPI Group (UK) Ltd, Croydon, CR0 4YY
Printed in North America by CPI GPS partners

We operate a distinctive and ethical publishing philosophy in
all areas of our business, from our global network of authors to
production and worldwide distribution.

Contents

Leaving the City

Health and Happiness in the Other America

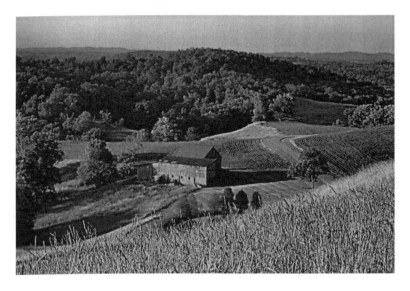

Dr Jeffrey A Tipton
Foreword by Dr Stephen Post
Author of Why Good Things Happen to Good People

Foreword

I lived in semi-rural Ohio for many years and I have lived in big and small cities and towns across America. I am very familiar with the landscape of this country. I am among those who think of Los Angeles or New York City as nice places for a business trip, but as a tad too stressful for everyday living. When I was living in my relatively small town in Ohio, I knew a great many people by name. I knew their children too and watched them grow up and head off to the big cities for college. In our neighborhood we could call out and invite a passerby up to the porch for casual conversation. We had real sidewalks, real neighborhood schools, and real love of neighbor and nature.

Dr. Jeffrey Tipton has written a visionary book about health and happiness in the "other" America – the places outside of the intense urban centers like NYC and LA. The urban world is known for its harried pace, mutual alienation, and distance from the rhythms of nature and of human nature. He focuses not merely on contagion, pollutants, violence, and innumerable other sources – both natural and human – of illness, disability, and premature death that one finds in urban America, but also addresses the inherent unhappiness and threats to mental health that life in the urban world typically brings. He contends, and rightly so, that those living in the big city have been robbed of the many joyful things life has to offer – community, connectedness and nature. He compares the earthy lives of our founders and philosophers like Emerson and Thoreau with the rather empty and disconnected lives of so many urbanites. He moves powerfully at the end of the book toward the emotional, relational, behavioral and self-reliance aspects of well-being that one can find in the "other America."

As Dr. Tipton highlights throughout the book, in the United States, self-reported happiness has been flat for decades, or

1

has even slightly declined since the late 1930s, despite each generation having more material wealth than did the preceding one. Anxiety and depression are up, especially among teens. While those whose basic material needs are met are happier than those who struggle in poverty, once basic needs are met, increased material prosperity does not bring increased happiness. This is in part because people tend to assess their level of relative prosperity by making comparisons with those who have more, and thus always perceive themselves as wanting. But it is also because financial capital does not equate with social capital. Americans today, while better off materially than their forebears, now report having only two very close friends, whereas twenty years ago they had three. This loss of "social capital," which occurs despite material prosperity, has been described with terms such as "bowling alone." The United States ranks 18th among nations in the 2020 "world map of happiness."

Living in a big city is clearly a risk factor for unhappiness. Researchers have now established the benefits to the agent of altruistic or "other-regarding" behavior in the domains of families, neighborhood, and society. If kind emotions and/or helping behavior are associated with well-being and health, we need to express these capacities. One finds that many urbanites have lost or never had much "other-regarding" behavior. Harvard's Pitirim A. Sorokin, in his classic 1954 treatise entitled, "The Ways and Power of Love", began his Preface with the assertion that unselfish love and altruism are "necessary for physical, mental, and moral health," and that "altruistic persons live longer than egoistic individuals." This connection has been examined in a major longitudinal prospective study of Harvard graduates over a fifty-year period, with the finding that generativity and happiness are very closely associated.

Well-being consists of feeling hopeful, happy and good about oneself, as well as energetic and connected to others.

Jeffrey Tipton describes current research on happiness and well-being, acknowledging that this is a complex area replete with confounders. But clearly "doing unto others," practicing "love of neighbor," and in general giving to others in heart and action is contributory to happiness. This is true for all ages. Stephanie Brown (2003), for example, reported on a five-year study involving 423 older couples. Each couple was asked what type of practical support they provided for friends or relatives, if they could count on help from others when needed, and what type of emotional support they gave each other. A total of 134 people died over the five years. After adjusting for a variety of factors – including age, gender, and physical and emotional health – the researchers found an association between reduced risk of dying and giving help, but no association between receiving help and reduced death risk. Brown, a researcher at the University of Michigan's Institute for Social Research, concluded that those who provided no instrumental or emotional support to others were more than twice as likely to die in the five years as people who helped spouses, friends, relatives, and neighbors. Despite concerns that the longevity effects might be due to a healthier individual's greater ability to provide help, the results remained the same after the researchers controlled for functional health, health satisfaction, health behaviors, age, income, education level, and other possible confounders. The researchers concluded that, "If giving, rather than receiving, promotes longevity, then interventions that are currently designed to help people feel supported may need to be redesigned so that the emphasis is on what people do to help others."

"Doing unto others" results in deeper and more positive social integration, distraction from personal problems and the anxiety of self-preoccupation, enhanced meaning and purpose as related to well-being, a more active lifestyle that counters cultural pressures toward isolated passivity, and the presence of positive emotions such as kindness that displace harmful negative emotional states. It is entirely quite plausible, then, to assert that altruism enhances happiness and health. The idea that human beings are inclined toward helpful pro-social and altruistic behavior seems incontrovertible, and it is highly plausible that the inhibition of such behavior and related emotions would be unhealthy.

The essential conclusion of this Foreword is that a strong association exists between the well-being, happiness, and health of people who are emotionally kind and compassionate in their charitable helping activities – as long as they are not overwhelmed, and here world view may come into play. The great challenge of urban living – and of living in general – is to live a generous life, which is also a happier and healthier one. The freedom from a solipsistic life in which one relates to others only in so far as they contribute to one's own agendas, as well as a general freedom from the narrow concerns of the self, bring us internal benefits, as all significant spiritual and moral traditions prescribe. Urban living, so often disconnected to others and self in so many ways, is not conducive to the neighborly ways one finds in less dense environments. And it is those neighborly ways that bring happiness.

Stephen G. Post, Ph.D.
Director, Center for Medical Humanities, Compassionate Care and Bioethics
Professor of Family, Population and Preventive Medicine
Stony Brook University

Introduction

All great and honorable actions are accompanied with great difficulties and must be both met and overcome with answerable courage.

~ William Bradford, *Of Plymouth Plantation*, 1651

We live in unprecedented times. Life has forever changed. Some of those changes are good and some are bad, some very bad. A little virus named COVID came along and put us in masks, locked in our homes, hurt us and killed us. COVID took the economy and spun it around and in many ways put it in a lockdown. But, as we all know, sometimes problems can end up being opportunities. If you ever contemplated changing your life then perhaps now is the time to do so since change is kind of the norm now. If you live in a big city and don't like it, then a cosmic porthole has opened up and this could be your chance to step to the other side. Leave the city.

There has been a bit of an exodus of people from big cities to smaller towns over the past five years. New York is actually losing population for the first time in forever. California lost around 200,000 people in 2020. While COVID has been a factor in this urban-to-rural migration, it was happening before the pandemic. U.S. census figures show that since 2014, an average of about 30,000 residents between 25 and 39 left big cities annually, but Americans of all ages and backgrounds are leaving them, especially those who live in New York and San Francisco. While a mass exodus from California clearly didn't happen in 2020, the pandemic did change some historical patterns. For example, "fewer people moved into the state to replace those who left," Natalie Holmes, research fellow at the California Policy Lab, said in a statement. "At the county level, however, San Francisco is experiencing a unique and dramatic exodus, which is causing 50% or 100% increases in Bay Area in-migration for some counties in the Sierras." Since the beginning of the pandemic, net domestic exits from the Bay Area "have increased 178% compared to pre-pandemic trends, with a 9% increase in departures and a 21% decrease in entrances in the last three quarters of 2020 relative to the same period in 2019," according to the study. During the last three quarters of 2020, San Francisco saw the largest percentage increase in residential exits of any county in the state, data shows. In the second through fourth quarters of 2020, exits from San Francisco "were 31% higher than during the same period in 2019." New entrances were 21% lower, the study said. Net exits from San Francisco in the last nine months of 2020 increased nearly 650% compared with the same period in 2019 – from 5,200 net exits to 38,800.

During this same time, small towns and cities in Texas, Utah, Arizona and Florida have doubled in population. A combination of COVID, economic disruption, civil disturbances and the move to remote work are clear factors in this *Green Acres* movement.

I cannot tell you what the ideal living environment is for you. All I can do is present you with facts, ideas, and some case studies of those who have left the big city and moved to small towns, farms, forests, a patch of dirt on a hill. Where you live influences your health. There is a growing understanding in the healthcare world that one's living environment influences health as much as genetics. Social determinants of health are the conditions in which people are born, grow, live, work and age. Your living environment – quality of housing, air, water, crime and access to open space – is something that needs to be considered.

The founders of this country were farmers, hunters and small business owners. They weren't great at any of it really when they first arrived, but they figured it out. And they had to cross the Atlantic, suffer through starvation and horrible diseases and throw off their British overlords to have the opportunity to get to this simple yet challenging life. For them, owning a piece of land and working it was akin to owning a slice of heaven.

The majority of Americans live in urban environments. About 50 million Americans live in the nation's rural counties, 200 million in suburbs and small metros and over 100 million in its urban core counties. Rural land makes up 97% of the land in this country yet only 18% of people live there.

The industrial revolution pulled people off their farms and led them to the fledgling cities and captured newly-arrived immigrants in the early 1900s. People have continued their march to or have been entrenched in urbania ever since... until now. In the mid and later 1900s there was growth of office jobs, growth of the suburbs, and a commuter class developed. Tech jobs became hot in the later part of the century, and before we knew it most of us had computers and cell phones and some of us started working from home. And America stopped being a manufacturing powerhouse. Factories died. We became a service and tech economy.

Things are radically different now than they were at the start of the 1900s. COVID, the civil disturbances of 2020, and other factors have pushed us even further into a new realm. Change in life is inevitable and expected. Radical change is disruptive. That's where we are now. We are at a jumping-off point. People are reevaluating their lives.

There is a psychological concept known as learned helplessness. The concept comes from the operant conditioning experiments done by Martin Seligman in the sixties at the University of Pennsylvania. In the experiments, Seligman set up a chamber where he put dogs with a barrier in the center. Every few minutes a light came on for 10 seconds, followed by a painful electric shock. The dog could escape the shock by jumping over the barrier; the dog could avoid the shock altogether by jumping over the barrier during the light presentation. Dogs learned to escape fairly quickly, and most learned to avoid the shock with extensive practice. Seligman then tried a different procedure with some new dogs. These animals were first restrained in a harness and given several light-shock pairings. Seligman thought that this might teach them the significance of the light as a signal for shock, and that this might encourage fast avoidance learning in the chamber. Unfortunately these dogs performed poorly in the chamber. When the light was presented they acted afraid. Although unrestrained, the animals lay on the floor and whimpered when the shock was presented. Seligman realized that the training with light and shock in the harness had taught these animals that they could not do anything about the delivery of shock. He called this phenomenon learned helplessness. According to Seligman, the key factor in the development of learned helplessness is the experience of having a lack of control over the environment.

2020 and 2021 delivered a series of devastating shocks that most of us were not able to avoid. Some of us tried to jump to the other side of the cage and others just lied down. Prior to the pandemic, many urbanites were already experiencing the cumulative trauma of the psychic shocks to the system one encounters in the big city. Many had been beaten down by traffic, noise, the high cost of living... the tyranny of bureaucracy. Then the pandemic hit, and the civil disturbances, the election, and the crumbling of the economy. For many, it was too much.

While the founders of this country were independent and self-reliant, most of us, and especially urbanites, live in a state of dependency. We rely on the delivery of water, food, power and that all important Internet for survival. Most of us don't know how to farm, fish, hunt, nor make a fire. If we were thrown in the woods naked most of us would die and not look pretty doing it. While some would argue that we have wisely outsourced the things our founders wasted their time doing such as growing their own food so we can spend more time in cerebral activities, the reality is we have become somewhat debilitated. What would you do if the water to your Manhattan condo was cut off? Call the city and complain? Go on Amazon and try to get some delivered? But what if you weren't the only one in this situation? Let's say there are millions of your close neighbors in this situation. Pandemonium would ensue. Many urbanites are becoming aware of the truly dependent state they're in and are moving to places where they have more control of their lives. Places where they fully understand where their water comes from and know exactly how to get some if the supply gets disrupted. Places where they can grow their own food if they so choose. Places where they become self-reliant. In control.

Many are now reconsidering how and where they live. After every major crisis, humanity is forced to identify those weaknesses and evolve accordingly. COVID and other 2020 evolutionary factors are responsible for the following changes and more in everyday life:

Around fifty percent of workers now work remotely. Millions left their offices in March and very few of them will return. For most Americans, you are now or will be able to live and work wherever you want.

Many jobs have become automated. There are self-driving cars on the road now. Your job, whatever it is, can be outsourced to a computer. At the start of 2020, were you worried a robot or computer was going to take over your job? If you weren't then you should be now. Imagine a way of life where you can't be replaced by a computer or robot and head towards that.

Shopping is largely done online now and that is not going to change. Have a job in a department store? It's going away. There's no great reason to live near great shops if all can be delivered to you.

Healthcare is being delivered electronically. Telemedicine was creeping along, but took serious hold during the pandemic.

Sure, a surgeon can't reach through your computer screen and take out your gallbladder, but so much can be done by phone and by screen. You don't need to live near Cedars to get Cedars level care.

Anxiety and depression are up three-fold. Students in particular have been hurt; they are sad, lonely and anxious. Best to live in an environment that is peaceful because this pandemic stressful existence is not going away soon.

Travel is a lot more difficult. There were less flights, more restrictions, more danger and less free little bags of peanuts. Many vacation places continue to be in various states of lockdown anyways and will be that way for a long time. The COVID vaccine could of course change a lot of that... til the next virus shows up.

Education will remain virtual. If you have kids, they will most likely be out of the classroom for a long time unless you live in a place where they don't care if kids get COVID. If you are in college, well you can choose to live where you want to do that and sit on the couch and get to work.

We live in pandemic times. A lot of people have been infected and get infected daily. Yes, there is a vaccine, but also new strains of the virus are occurring constantly. Your fellow humans harbor viruses that can kill you. The more of them you are near the higher chance you will become infected. The less people you come in contact with the better.

In the chapters ahead, I will detail the threats to health and happiness in urban America; describe life in the other America; provide some case studies of those who left the big city and thrived; and finally provide a guide to help you make your own *Green Acres* move if you choose to do so. As before, I can't tell you where to live. The "soul" purpose of this book is to provide facts about how and where we Americans live while comparing how we were living at the country's founding and where we have now landed. I am, of course, making a case for another and quite possibly a better way of life outside of the big city. If you hate traffic, noise, crowds and rude people... well, you don't have to put up with it... there's another America.

And finally, I'll get personal. Eight years ago I started a nonprofit after spending a few years advocating for rehabilitation of the beat-down LA River and turning it into a recreational zone. For eight years, I helped many people get down a small section of the LA River near downtown. I and the people who participated thoroughly enjoyed themselves. Before the summer of 2020, I was informed by the City of LA that kayaking was not to be allowed as participants could possibly be exposed to COVID while kayaking – not exactly sure how that would happen as the kayaks are one-person. The City of LA then offered to allow me to do virtual kayaking – put people on rented rowing machines in their homes, but no rental rowing machines were available because of COVID-related demand for rental exercise equipment. I offered to buy the rowing machines and give them to participants, but was told by the City that they did not want the liability. In the summer of 2020, I also received notice from the California Franchise Tax Board that my nonprofit status was being revoked because a clerk there believed that my nonprofit was actually a kayak rental business and that I should be paying taxes on the 5,000 a year or so dollars that participants paid for the experience of kayaking down the LA River that I had opened up for recreational use. All participants received education about the history of the LA River and kayak instruction when necessary. I took no salary from the program and donated my time and money to make it run. My nonprofit was in good standing with the IRS as a 501I(3) and all state fees had been paid. After a three-month surreal battle with the Franchise Tax Board, they decided they were wrong and reinstated my nonprofit exempt status. Shortly after this experience with the City of LA and the Franchise Tax Board and many other stupefying

LA and State of California experiences, I decided enough was enough. I bought some property in Missouri and Florida and left California and the City of Fallen Angels behind. I was born in LA, grew up in Santa Barbara, and then returned to live in LA for some 30 years. While I was sad to leave LA, the beat down had become too much. If you live in urban America, how many horror tales of soul crushing bureaucracy do you have? How many hours of mind-numbing traffic? Parking tickets that represent a significant portion of your income? You don't have to endure it. There is another life. I hope you enjoy the read ahead.

Chapter 1

Living

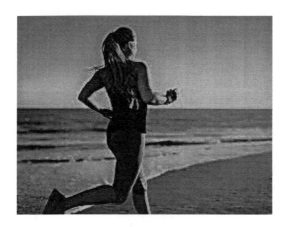

Living Defined

The ultimate value of life depends upon awareness, and the power of contemplation rather than upon mere survival.

~ Aristotle

Those who have lived in big cities or visited them, know they can be pressure cookers – true Darwinian jungles, survival of the fittest laboratories. Freeway chases that end in death are actually a form of entertainment in some cities. With city living comes some unique struggles for survival. For example, you have people from all over the world living and visiting cities and they can bring some unique diseases, like COVID, with them. Cities can also be gang infested and polluted. And terrorists have brought another survival threat to big cities.

At the most basic level, staying alive is living. For some urban residents, just making it through the day without getting shot is an accomplishment. Most U.S. urbanites, however, are not engaged in a life and death struggle every day. Most have roofs over their heads; food to eat; some air to breathe; and some water to drink. Many urbanites these days are at least "surviving" on a basic level. When people say, "I'm surviving," however, they are usually describing a situation where they are barely holding their head above water. Most people yearn for more than just "survival." Sure, many urbanites are surviving, but they are not thriving, and with COVID, well, that has changed everything.

Lifetime odds of death for selected causes, United States[1]

Cause of Death	Odds of Dying
Heart disease	1 in 6
Cancer	1 in 7
All preventable causes of death	1 in 25
Chronic lower respiratory disease	1 in 26
Suicide	1 in 86
Opioid overdose	1 in 98
Motor-vehicle crash	1 in 106
Fall	1 in 111
Gun assault	1 in 298
Pedestrian incident	1 in 541
Motorcyclist	1 in 890
COVID	1 in 1,000*
Drowning	1 in 1,121
Fire or smoke	1 in 1,399
Choking on food	1 in 2,618
Bicyclist	1 in 4,054
Accidental gun discharge	1 in 9,077
Sharp objects	1 in 29,483
Hot surfaces and substances	1 in 45,186
Hornet, wasp, and bee stings	1 in 53,989
Cataclysmic storm	1 in 54,699

Dog attack	1 in 118,776
Lightning	1 in 180,746
Railway passenger	Too few deaths in 2018 to calculate odds
Passenger on an airplane	Too few

*COVID odds are for period from 12/20 to 06/21

COVID increased the overall risk of death for the average American by about 10%, but this increase in risk was much higher for seniors than children. For seniors age 70 and older, getting COVID is riskier than climbing Mt. Everest; in contrast, for those under age 20, the infection fatality risk is equivalent to driving a car for 7,500 miles. One in 12 people who attempt to climb Mt. Everest die. If you're over 80 then you are 20 times likely to die from COVID than someone in their fifties.[2]

Prior to the COVID pandemic, it seemed that living was a bit of a given – life was being taken for granted. The provision of basic needs is now a reasonable expectation in developed countries and people generally expect good health as well. Due to improvements in medicine, public health, and nutrition, life expectancy has gone up and has done so dramatically during the past one hundred years. Life expectancy at birth in the United States in 1901 was 49 years. At the end of the twentieth century life expectancy reached 77 years, an increase of greater than 50% in one hundred years.[3]

Humans by Era, Average Lifespan (in years):[4]

Neanderthal, 20
Neolithic, 20
Classical Greece, 28
Classical Rome, 28
Medieval England, 33
End of 18th Century, 37

Early 20th Century, 50

1940, 65

Current (in the West), 84

While people are living longer and healthier lives, there are still many threats to survival. Many have forgotten that in the past century millions of people were killed as a result of two World Wars. The influenza pandemic of 1918-19 alone killed more than 21 million people worldwide, AIDS is still killing people, COVID has killed and debilitated millions. It is likely that COVID will be the leading cause of death in the U.S. in 2020. Many wars are still being fought around the globe and a variety of other infectious diseases kill many people every day. The world's population continues to expand (nearly eight billion) and resources continue to shrink. Weather extremes are occurring; new bugs are showing up every year; and world peace has not been declared. Life is still fairly uncertain.

"Living" for the purposes of this book is as much about finding satisfaction or happiness as it is about staying alive, because in the end most feel they are "living" when all of their needs are being met. Most people, however, seem to need more than a functioning heart, a place to live, and three square meals to feel satisfied. Some believe that they are not truly living if they don't have a new car every year. Many believe that if they simply had a lot of money they would find satisfaction. A classic study by happiness researcher Ed Diener, however, which compared the happiness of multimillionaires (incomes over $10 million a year) to a group of middle income earners (who made on average $36,000), found that the super wealthy were only slightly happier overall.[5] Money is not the key to happiness, but it is certainly necessary for getting needs met.

So what does it take for a person to feel satisfied or happy? It depends on the person, but most at least expect what the framers of the Constitution promised: life, liberty and the pursuit of happiness. People want to be happy, but what do people need to feel happy? Happiness or satisfaction can be a very subjective thing, yet there seem to be some common ingredients in the mix. Few feel satisfied if they are not getting their basic needs met and most people aren't happy when they are physically ill. Many people feel dissatisfied if they are not getting their material or ego needs met. And many feel deprived if they are not engaged in meaningful relationships with others. Happiness is in the end a very subjective thing; everyone has their own way to float their boat, but most of us certainly know the things that make us unhappy.

Satisfaction

Meaning is experienced by the self-actualized, growth-motivated person who delights in using their creative powers for their own sake, and who can affirm themself and simultaneously transcend through peak experiences.

~ Abraham Maslow

Noted psychologist Abraham Maslow tried to capture this elusive phenomenon of human satisfaction in the 1950s. He established the theory of a hierarchy of needs, writing that humans are motivated by unsatisfied needs, and that certain lower needs need to be satisfied before higher needs can be satisfied. The basic premise is that people are need-driven organisms, and if they don't have their needs met then they don't feel satisfied and are unhappy. According to Maslow, and basic logic, there are general types of needs (physiological, safety, love, esteem) that must be satisfied before a person can move up the needs ladder. While this movement toward self-actualization is not necessarily an orderly process, we generally look to satisfy higher needs after our lower needs are met.[6] For example, if an individual's life or physical safety were suddenly threatened while they were dining, they would probably stop their conversation about global warming and run. People routinely interrupt other activities to respond to the promptings of hunger, thirst, fatigue, discomfort or pain, or a physical threat. There are also many interactions among our needs; they are not independent. And, of course, there are many potential conflicts between our needs. The obvious examples are situations where one's safety might have to be jeopardized in order to obtain food or other necessities, or where one's personal nutrition, health, and safety needs might have to be sacrificed for the sake of a family member. In the end, it seems that people are "needs junkies" who have to get their "fixes" in order to feel happy or satisfied. When a person's total needs aren't met they become physically ill or depressed or both.

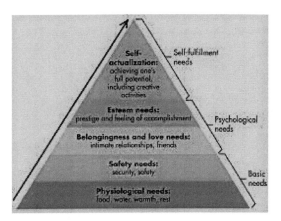

Physiological Needs

Physiological needs are the very basic needs: the need for air, water, food, elimination, sleep, and sex. If a person's physiological needs aren't met then they die. Physiological needs are primal and motivate people to alleviate such needs as soon as possible; a person can't really think about much else until their physiological needs are met. If a person is tired or hungry or thirsty then they typically put all else on hold. In other words, a person is probably not going to spend much time thinking about how to help starving children in Africa if they haven't had anything to eat for a few days.

Most adults need between 1,500 and 2,500 hundred calories (kcal) of energy a day to satisfy basic energy needs and around 64 ounces of water – you can only live a few days without water and some can last weeks without food. There is debate about how much sleep people need, but eight hours per night is often noted as ideal. Exact food requirements are often debated – ask several nutritionists what the ideal diet is and they'll give different answers. And an appropriate quantity of calories is not the only variable to consider: people also need to consider if they are getting enough essential elements, fiber and the like. Conversely, it is also possible to consume too many calories – over-consumption of sugars, fats and overdoses of certain vitamins being especially notable problems today.[7] And the quality of air, water and food is another concern. People devote significant resources to get their physiological needs met. Most Americans assume that their basic physiological needs will be met, and they get pretty upset when they are cut off from regular sources of water and food. Life, as most Americans know it, would essentially come to a stop if, for example, the water supply were to be suddenly and irreversibly contaminated. One can imagine how difficult it would be to continue working or studying in the context of an extended denial of such primary needs as sleep, food, water, or waste elimination. A great percentage of life is devoted to making sure physiological needs are met even if it seems that people don't spend much time thinking about it.

Safety Needs

People need stability and consistency. People need to feel safe and secure. People want a predictable world. Unfortunately, when one thinks of city life images of stability and consistency don't pop up. COVID, that little thing you can't see, has rattled the predictability of life. Like other needs, people's safety needs differ; some have more safety needs than others. There are some who feel they need to have a gun to feel safe; others feel they need to live in a gated or guarded community to be safe. Some need the security of a home and family to feel safe, and others don't. People generally want law and order; they want to be able to go for a walk in their neighborhood without getting mugged. Some people leave the big city because they have concluded that the city is simply not a safe place to live. And terrorism is a definite urban safety concern. Terrorists like to blow up big buildings; they don't blow up farms. Things have been somewhat quiet on that front for a while, but that threat is not going away.

Belonging Needs

We humans are social beings. We come into the world as the result of others' actions. We survive here in dependence on others. Whether we like it or not, there is hardly a moment of our lives when we do not benefit from others' activities. For this reason it is hardly surprising that most of our happiness arises in the context of our relationships with others.

~ HH the Dalai Lama

Belonging or love needs are next on Maslow's pyramid. Humans have a need to belong to groups: clubs, work groups, religious groups, and family. People need to feel loved (nonsexual) by others and to be accepted by others. People need to be needed; they want to "belong." While some human social activity may be born of personal preservation, some of it seems to be related to societal preservation; humans seem to care about the survival of other humans too. Maslow described these belonging needs as follows:[8]

If both the physiological and the safety needs are fairly well gratified, then there will emerge the love and affection and belongingness needs, and the whole cycle already described will repeat itself with this new center. Now the person will feel keenly, as never before, the absence of friends, or a sweetheart, or a wife, or children. He will hunger for affectionate relations with people in general, namely, for a place in his group, and he will strive with great intensity to achieve this goal. He will want to attain such a place more than anything else in the world and may even forget that once, when he was hungry, he sneered at love.

Esteem Needs

Maslow noted two versions of esteem needs, a lower one and a higher one. The lower one is the need for the respect of others, the need for status, fame, glory, recognition, attention, reputation, appreciation, dignity, even dominance. The higher form involves the need for self-respect, including such feelings as confidence, competence, achievement, mastery, independence, and freedom. It seems that humans have a need for a stable, firmly based, high level of self-respect, and respect from others. When these needs are satisfied, the person feels self-confident and valuable as a person in the world. People need to feel that they are special and they need to hear about it from others. When esteem needs are frustrated, the person feels inferior, weak, helpless and worthless. Maslow felt that the negative versions of these esteems – low self-esteem and inferiority complex – were at the root of most psychological problems.

Self-Actualization

Try not to become a man of success but rather become a man of value.
~ Albert Einstein

According to Maslow, self-actualization is the desire to become more and more what one is, and to become everything that one is capable of becoming. Once people have most of their other needs met they often focus on the need of maximizing their human potential. They seek knowledge, peace, esthetic experiences, self-fulfillment, and delve into the spiritual. They relax their ego needs, and explore and enjoy life, and think beyond their own needs. Self-actualized people find satisfaction in caring for others and for finding a greater meaning in life. Self-actualization is a state where one finds trust in an ultimate reality; a state of self-awareness in which fears and desires have been transcended, and a person has consciously chosen values.

It seems that in order to feel truly satisfied a person needs to find a balance of satisfying the needs of others and their own needs. It rings true that when a person only seeks to satisfy the self and not contribute to relationships or society they can feel alienated from others and the world. Likewise, when people commit themselves to personal relationships, society or work, and neglect their individual selves, they also feel dissatisfied. And clearly, if a person feels they can find total satisfaction in the material world they will ultimately be disappointed.

He who does not tire, tires adversity.

~ Anonymous

Living then it seems is as much about staying alive as it is about flourishing and finding some kind of inner peace. At the most basic level one needs their health to survive. To maintain health a person needs quality food, water, air, safe shelter, healthcare, exercise and rest. Some of the aforementioned can be had with little or no money, but the reality is that people need money to survive, especially in big city environments. The amount of money one needs is determined by what their needs are, but most people can survive on less than they think they need.

People also need loving relationships or at least some healthy connection to others; people don't fare well in isolation. On the personal development front one needs to determine what gives their life meaning – if a person feels that being a lifeguard is their life's purpose then they should become a lifeguard. And, as Maslow and others have discovered, the things that perhaps bring the most satisfaction are the things a person does to benefit others and the world in general. People greatly benefit from connection to others. Unfortunately, in big cities, there may be a lot of people, but very few true connections to others.

Self-Reliance

Nothing can bring you peace but yourself.
~ Ralph Waldo Emerson

And finally, a bit on the concept of self-reliance and its relationship to living and happiness. Self-reliance has many components, but at its most basic level it is, "Can you take care of yourself?" and at its more abstract level, "Are your thoughts truly your own?" Think back to when you were a baby (that memory is in there somewhere) and what it felt like to take your first steps: quite an accomplishment! That was for you, by you. Now think of yourself standing in line to get a five dollar latte at Starbucks. Does that feel as powerful as your first steps? Sure, you worked hard (or not) for that five dollars, but you are outsourcing your beverage needs and paying dearly for it. Noted philosopher Ralph Waldo Emerson pontificated on self-reliance in his eponymous 1841 essay "Self-Reliance." The essay advocated for not following societal norms and conventions as they take away from getting to know thyself. He contended that no one becomes a leader by being a follower. How many layers of society and familial expectations have been laid down on you over the years? Where is that baby that took those steps?

Exercising self-reliance is a great way to increase self-confidence which in turn fortifies you with a sense of security. The more you act in a self-reliant way – fix your own toilet, grow your own food – the more certain you become of your own abilities. By building your self-reliance, you can trust yourself to rely on your own internal resources. Practicing your self-reliance helps you overcome obstacles, learn from failures, and impact your own self-worth and self-confidence. Sure, there is still room to have others in your life, but you will feel better when you have the tools to do it alone. You are not truly living if you depend on others for your existence.

To finish this chapter, I conclude with a video link from the Modern Self Reliance channel on YouTube. In it, brothers Kevin and Chris enthusiastically talk about what they are building on a plot of land in the woods with the goal of being completely self-sufficient. They aren't wilderness professionals, just two regular guys figuring out how to live. I'm sure if there were cameras back in the days of our founders, you'd see something similar. Figuring how to auto-pay your LA Department of Water and Power bill is not an accomplishment. Figuring out how to bring water and electricity into the home you built is. A smaller life is totally obtainable and ultimately can make your life bigger in ways unimaginable.

What is Modern Self Reliance: https://youtu.be/n7m0Cdt4f8Y

Chapter 2

The Rise of the Big City

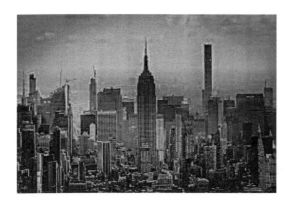

The City Defined

Civilizations die from suicide, not by murder.
~ Arnold Toynbee

Cities, as living environments, are unique and hold unique threats to one's physical and mental well-being. When one thinks "city" a few things immediately come to mind: tall buildings, traffic, and lots of people. Cities are built environments with large and dense populations, but there is more to cities than skyscrapers and crowds. Lewis Mumford, an early twentieth century city historian and the author of *The Culture of Cities* (1937), described the city as a symphony.[9] Arnold Toynbee, the British economist, described cities in more functionalist terms as "a cluster of buildings with a dense population unable to raise its own food but able to supply goods and services to those in the country in exchange for food."[10] Cities consist of both social and physical phenomena; they are form, function, and ideals. Cities are typically regional centers of government and commerce. Cities have museums, libraries, universities, sports and entertainment venues; they have a culture. And on the flipside, cities can be plagued with crime, disasters, infectious diseases, social unrest, and pollution. Cities often represent the best and worst of humankind. Cities are, by definition, legal entities of any size where a large number of people live. Demographers, urban sociologists, urban geographers and the like have, of course, further defined the city. Within cities there are downtowns and uptowns; exurbs and boomburgs; edge cities and inner cities. And in some regions of the country – the Northeast, California – the cities have simply merged and become one large city (a megalopolis). The megalopolis known as BosWash extends from Boston to Washington DC; the SanSan megalopolis starts in San Francisco and ends in San Diego.[11]

The city, for the purpose of this book, is best exemplified by U.S. cities like New York, Chicago, Los Angeles, and Houston; cities may not be easy to define, but most know one if they see one. While U.S. cities are certainly not exactly alike, they do share some common elements: large, diverse, and dense populations; a largely built environment, and a particular culture.

The March to Urbanization

Over the next two decades the majority of the world's population will live in urban areas and the number of urban residents in developing countries will double, increasing by over 2 billion inhabitants. In the 1800s, 97% of the world's population was rural, and now it is estimated that over 70% of the population is urban. The earliest cities were founded near rivers and were often centers of worship. Jericho, a stone-walled cluster of mud buildings that housed several thousand people around 8000 BCE, and Catalhoyuk, an even larger settlement of mud buildings in Anatolia (Turkey), were some of the world's earliest cities. It is generally agreed that cities came into existence as a result of agricultural development and mastering of animal husbandry, the so-called agricultural revolution. Improvements in agriculture gave people some "free time" and allowed them to get involved in other endeavors; cities developed as a result of excess. Before the beginning of the Common Era, Rome, Constantinople, and Chinese and Indian capitals had populations of a half million and more. Rome flourished from the first century BCE, until it was ultimately conquered and divided in the fifth century. By the fifth century the population of Rome had been reduced to 250,000 from nearly one million inhabitants at its peak.[12] Edward Gibbon, the author of *The History of the Decline and Fall of the Roman Empire*, concluded that the Roman Empire succumbed to barbarian invasions because of a loss of civic virtue among its citizens. Romans had become lazy and soft, entrusting their duties to defend their Empire to barbarian mercenaries. According to Gibbon, the Romans had become effeminate and were unwilling to live the military lifestyle. He also implicated Christianity in the downfall of Rome. Gibbon believed that Christianity created a belief in another world and suggested that a better life existed after death.[13]

By 1500 only some two dozen places in the world contained more than 100,000 inhabitants; as late as 1700 there were still fewer than 40 – the black plague and incessant wars dramatically reduced urban populations. The growth of modern industry from the late 18th century onward led to massive urbanization and the rise of new great cities, first in Europe and then in other regions, as new opportunities brought huge numbers of migrants from rural communities into urban areas. By 1900 there were more than 300 cities in the world with populations greater than 100,000.[14]

United States Urbanization

Eight of the 10 largest metropolitan areas in the United States developed in the 19th century.[15] In 1790, 94% of the U.S. population lived in the countryside. After 1830 the urban areas of the country grew more rapidly than the rural areas. By 1890, industrialization coupled with substantial immigration had produced substantial growth in cities, and 35% of Americans lived in urban areas, mostly in the northern half of the United States. The number of Americans living in cities did not surpass the number in rural areas until 1920. By the 1990s three out of four Americans lived in an urban setting.

Suburbs began to appear in the 18th century as wealthy people built second homes in the country to escape the crowded, sweltering city during the summer. A few began living outside the city full-time and commuting by carriage to town. Commuting into the city to work became easier and cheaper in the late 19th century when commuter railroad lines were built, radiating out from the central city. As the suburbs grew, more and more of the middle classes abandoned the cities. The suburbs were attractive for many reasons: they were cleaner, newer, had better-funded schools, were socially homogeneous, and provided a sense of security.[16] A lot of those early suburbs are now big cities and people are leaving them to move to the new suburbs – the exurbs.

In 2000, 80% of Americans (226 million people) lived in metropolitan areas. Western and Southern cities have grown the fastest, while urban industrial centers in the Midwest and Northeast have actually declined in population. New York continues to be the country's largest and most densely populated city. Overall, cities expanded rapidly during the 1990s, growing nearly twice as fast as in the 1980s. While most U.S. cities continue to grow, the pace is slower and a lot of current growth reflects the changing demographics; the U.S. is becoming a country of retirees, and a lot of retired folks are moving to where the sun is. Although some cities have experienced a downtown renaissance of sorts, immigration still accounts for most inner city or downtown growth.[17] In the end, most Americans seem to prefer to live outside of the city and people like nice weather and that's where the growth is.

Population of America's 10 Largest Cities

		2019	2010	Increase
1	New York City	8,336,817	8,175,133	+1.98%
2	Los Angeles	3,979,576	3,792,621	+4.93%
3	Chicago	2,693,976	2,695,598	−0.06%
4	Houston	2,320,268	2,100,263	+10.48%
5	Phoenix	1,680,992	1,445,632	+16.28%
6	Philadelphia	1,584,064	1,526,006	+3.80%
7	San Antonio	1,547,253	1,327,407	+16.56%
8	San Diego	1,423,851	1,307,402	+8.91%
9	Dallas	1,343,573	1,197,816	+12.17%
10	San Jose	1,021,795	945,942	+8.02%

The Difference a City Makes

Due to city size people cannot possibly know all other urbanites. Out of necessity, there is a shift away from primary relationships to secondary relationships. Urbanites interact with others not as individuals but with others in certain roles. For example, an urban dweller deals with many people in the course of the day such as the deli cashier and the doorman of his or her apartment building. The urbanite does not develop deep personal connections with these people but only interacts with them in terms of their roles. Personal relations become superficial and transitory. Urban life is marked by utilitarianism and efficiency. The density of living and heterogeneity of urban residents leads people to live in homogenous groups resulting in a "mosaic of social worlds" in a city. Transitions across groups are difficult, and numerous social orders result adding to the segmentation of urban life.

~ Louis Wirth, "Urbanism as a Way of Life," 1938

City life can differ dramatically from life in suburbia or rural life. An urbanite's standard of living is often higher than that of a rural dweller as a result of better employment opportunities, higher incomes and easier access to social and urban services. Cities, however, typically have higher violent crime rates; higher teen pregnancy rates; higher high school dropout rates; and higher rates of infant mortality than other living environs.[18] Using a statistical apples to apples comparison of sorts, it seems that life in Apple Creek, Ohio – a small town of 1,200 in the middle of Ohio – is not quite the same as life in the Big Apple. An Apple Creek resident is more likely than a New Yorker to be married with kids; to pay far less for housing; and to own their own home. Compared to the "Little Apple," New Yorkers are at higher risk of being victims of violent crime; they have a much longer commute to work; and they are exposed to more pollutants. Apple Creek is one of the safest places to live in America, and New York is in the lower 20th percentile.

Cities typically have dense populations – they are crowded – and crowding seems to change social dynamics. Researchers in the social sciences have long tried to explain the effects of urbanization on humans. Experiments done by Yale psychologist Stanley Milgram in the seventies suggest that when people are confronted with a large number of strangers in everyday life, they tend to withdraw and take less interest in the community in order to protect themselves from overload.[19] Other studies have shown that people withdraw or become aggressive when environs become too crowded.[20]

The urban environment – air, water, weather, and terrain – also differs from non-urban settings. Cities tend to be more polluted than other environs. This pollution results both from the concentration of population and from the way in which individuals and businesses act towards controlling potential sources of pollution. As the population grows, so often do the environmental problems. Large population concentration usually requires higher costs per person for the maintenance of clean water and the safe removal of garbage. Air quality, in particular, may be difficult to maintain at high population densities if there is not a natural flow of air through the area. Some cities, such as Los Angeles that is in a basin, have problems dealing with air quality because air is often trapped. City water, while heavily regulated, is another important urban issue. Deteriorating waterworks, pollution, and outdated treatment technology combine to deliver drinking water that is potentially unsafe. And foul weather can be especially foul for city dwellers. Cities often run a few degrees warmer and it is not uncommon for people to die during summer heat waves. The Katrina disaster also demonstrated how quickly things go wrong when a city is hit by a weather-related calamity – the population of New Orleans declined 200,000 people after the hurricane hit. And for places like Los Angeles, there is always the threat of an earthquake. If a magnitude eight earthquake was to hit Los Angeles – a realistic notion – thousands of people would die and the city would be decimated.

There is a perception that living in the city can be dangerous and statistics support this notion. Violent and property crime victimization disproportionately affected urban residents. In addition to the criminals and gang members that commit violent crimes on a regular basis in U.S. cities, foreign terrorists are also interested in hurting city dwellers. 2,986 people were killed – most in NYC – as a result of the September 11, 2001 attacks. In addition to those who lost their lives, many more were injured and the U.S. economy was devastated. While big city violent crime rates have gone down somewhat recently and there hasn't been a major terrorist attack in years, urban environs tend to be more violent than the "burbs."

Did You Know?

Motor vehicle theft occurs 2.2 times more frequently in urban areas than rural areas.

City life can also be stressful and unhealthy. Stress is an unrelenting fact of life in most cities. Most urbanites work at maximum capacity to meet expenses (in Manhattan the basics cost a family of four around $150,000 a year), and money and other worries push many to the edge and some over it – the heart attack rate in New York City is higher than the national average.[21] While most in the city die from what kills most in the U.S., living in the city can make it difficult to exercise and do other things one needs to do to stay healthy, and long commutes are especially unhealthy. Lack of access to healthcare can be another concern – so difficult sometimes to get that doctor's appointment. If a person has good insurance or a lot of money then they can usually find good care in the big city, but if they don't then they are often out of luck.

Cities have been a part of human existence for thousands of years. Cities have come and gone and thrived and withered throughout recorded history. With real estate sales way down in New York and other cities, it seems this is a withering moment. City living – lots of people jammed into a largely human-made environment – can be very stimulating, but lots of people living in close proximity to each other can also lead to problems and such problems are addressed in the chapters that follow.

Chapter 3

The Urban Environment

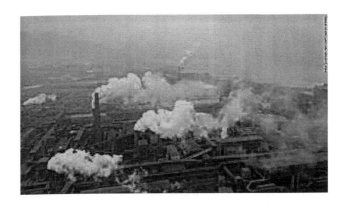

How long can men thrive between walls of brick, walking on asphalt pavements, breathing the fumes of coal and of oil, growing, working, dying, with hardly a thought of wind, and sky, and fields of grain, seeing only machine-made beauty, the mineral-like quality of life?

~ Charles A. Lindbergh, *Reader's Digest*, November 1939

There are many environmental factors that adversely impact human health or the ecological balances essential to long-term human health and environmental quality, whether in the natural or man-made environment. The environment – air, water, soil, weather, and to some degree the constructed habitats people live and work in – can profoundly influence health. For example, it is estimated that around 50,000 people per year die in the U.S. as a result of exposure to toxic agents in the environment. Urban environmental issues range from the personal – living with someone who smokes, to the far reaching, like a contaminated municipal water supply. The environmental quality of a city can have a dramatic effect on the health status of all residents – even the rich can't escape the effects of poor air and water quality, inadequate sanitation, a lack of proper solid waste management, and the improper storage and emission of hazardous substances. And while there are many known and obvious environmental concerns like lead and smog, there are many other things that are still being discovered.

Many cities are known for their persistent pollution problems, smoggy LA and Houston, and over the years there have been numerous environmental events (hurricanes, earthquakes, fires, tsunamis) to remind us how the environment can dramatically impact life. Cities are for the most part human-made habitats, and living off the concrete markedly differs from living off the land. And even though cities are largely built environments there are plenty of "natural" things in the environment that can also make city living difficult – city folks can suffer from plain old seasonal allergies too.

The World Health Organization's *Millennium Ecosystem Assessment* showed that some 60% of the benefits that the global ecosystem provides to support life on earth such as fresh water, clean air and a relatively stable climate are being degraded or used unsustainably. The report warned that harmful consequences of this degradation to human health are already being felt and could grow significantly worse over the next 50 years.[22] There is much concern about global warming as the mean global temperature has risen a few degrees over the past century and experts predict that this temperature rise will lead to massive environmental problems. The environment and how it impacts you is very real... you can't necessarily escape it in your air conditioned condo in Chicago. If sea levels rise and you live in a densely populated coastal city, your building could end up under water in the near future.

The environment truly is becoming a problem and urbanites are not only at risk of being harmed by the environment, they are also responsible for a lot of the world's environmental problems. Over the past two decades many have been striving to get a "handle" on the environment; there is a real fear that our planet is quickly deteriorating. The 2015 Paris Accord seeks to curb global warming. The accord calls for limiting the global average temperature rise in this century to well below two degrees Celsius. Participant countries are to level off greenhouse gas emissions as soon as possible and to become carbon neutral no later than the second half of this century. To achieve these objectives, participating countries responsible for more than 90% of global emissions submitted carbon reduction targets. These targets outlined each country's commitments for curbing emissions through 2030, including both economy-wide carbon-cutting goals and the individual commitments of some 2,250 cities and 2,025 companies.[23]

Such efforts reflect a growing understanding of the far-reaching effects that the environment can have on people's lives, especially urbanites. They also reflect an understanding that everyone contributes to the world's environmental problems on some level and that everyone can do something to improve the environment. If you are a commuter in a gas-powered car driving from your suburban home to the city then you are contributing to the problem.

Urban Air

Thank God men cannot fly, and lay waste the sky as well as the earth.
~ Henry David Thoreau

Air pollution is a major concern and a problem for many U.S. city dwellers. While some air pollution is obvious – a person can see, smell or taste the bad air – many air pollutants aren't obvious; even though a car may not look like it isn't spewing out pollutants it actually is. Air is essential for life, and bad air can ruin the quality of life and even shorten it. People breathe air every minute of every day. According to the EPA, an average person breathes in 3,400 gallons of air per day. Breathing then is a continuous route of exposure to potentially harmful agents. Compared with other things in the environment such as water and food, individuals have far less control over the quality of the air they breathe. This continuous exposure, lack of control, and possible negative health outcomes from exposure to poor quality air makes air quality an important environmental health issue. Even though the air is cleaner of late, smog continues to be a serious public health threat. It is estimated that around 24,000 people die each year in the U.S. as a result of air pollution.[24] The effect of air pollution on children is particularly striking. The World Health Organization published an in-depth look at the research on children's health and air pollution, and concluded that air pollution is directly responsible for some infant deaths. In addition, they found that air pollution caused other harm to children that included: short-term and long-term decreased lung function rates; aggravation of asthma; increased rates of cough and bronchitis; and increased rates of upper respiratory infections.[25] Urban children have much higher rates of asthma compared to their non-urban counterparts.

Air pollution is a broad term applied to any chemical, physical, or biological agent that modifies the natural characteristics of the atmosphere. Outdoor air pollution can be due to particulate matter (dust, diesel exhaust) and noxious gases such as sulfur dioxide, carbon monoxide, nitrogen oxides, and chemical vapors. These noxious gases take part in further chemical reactions once they are in the atmosphere forming smog and acid rain. The two primary pollutants in smog are ground-level ozone (O_3) and particulate matter (PM).[26] The greatest source of air pollution is the internal combustion engine – automobiles and trucks contribute up to 50% of the smog and 90% of the carbon monoxide in urban areas.[27] Although automobiles built today pollute less than those made in the 1960s, the increase in the total number of vehicles and urban sprawl have largely negated the benefit of improved technology. Other sources of ambient air pollution include generating stations, factories, office buildings, fires and dry cleaning facilities.

Indoor air pollution can be, of course, as deleterious as outdoor air pollution. Indoor air pollutants include such things as tobacco smoke, paint, and mold.

Exposure to air pollution has a number of health effects for humans and animals, and it harms plants and destroys property. As with any environmental exposure, the effects depend on the concentration, duration, and frequency of the exposure. Because people breathe in air pollutants through the lungs, many of the health effects occur in the pulmonary system. Different groups of individuals are affected by air pollution in different ways; some individuals are much more sensitive to pollutants than are others. Exposure to smog has been implicated in a range of illnesses and conditions, from asthma to pneumonia, from hay fever to sinusitis, and can trigger or aggravate cancer and emphysema. Young children and elderly people often suffer more from the effects of air pollution than others. People with health problems such as asthma, heart and lung disease also suffer more when the air is polluted. Short-term, high-level exposures to smog typically result in decreased lung function and upper respiratory irritation, but they can also be immediately fatal.[28] London experienced a very severe air pollution episode in 1952 that resulted in 4,000 deaths.[29] That was a long time ago, but air pollution extreme events still happen. The Bhopal Disaster of 1984 was caused by the accidental release of methyl isocyanate (MIC) from a Union Carbide pesticide plant located in the heart of the city of Bhopal, in the Indian state of Madhya Pradesh. The gases injured anywhere from 150,000 to 600,000 people, and killed 15,000.[30]

Long-term exposure to polluted air can increase rates of pulmonary infections and chronic bronchitis. And certain air pollutants have specific systemic toxic effects on the cardiovascular system. Continual exposure to air pollution stunts the growth of the lungs of children and may aggravate medical conditions in the elderly.[31] And let's not forget about one of the most harmful long-term air pollutants around, tobacco smoke. Smoking leads to disease and disability, and harms nearly every organ of the body. More than 16 million Americans are living with a disease caused by smoking. For every person who dies because of smoking, at least 30 people live with a serious smoking-related illness. Smoking causes cancer, heart disease, stroke, lung diseases, diabetes, and chronic obstructive pulmonary disease (COPD), which includes emphysema and chronic bronchitis. Smoking also increases risk for tuberculosis, certain eye diseases, and problems of the immune system, including rheumatoid arthritis. Secondhand smoke exposure contributes to approximately 41,000 deaths among nonsmoking adults and 400 deaths in infants each year. Secondhand smoke causes stroke, lung cancer, and coronary heart disease in adults. Children who are exposed to secondhand smoke are at increased risk for sudden infant death syndrome, acute respiratory infections, middle ear disease, more severe asthma, respiratory symptoms, and slowed lung growth. In 2019, nearly 14 of every 100 U.S. adults aged 18 years or older (14.0%) currently smoked cigarettes. This means an estimated 34.1 million adults in the United States currently smoke cigarettes. An estimated 58 million Americans – including 14 million children ages 3 to 11 – are exposed to secondhand smoke from cigarettes and other tobacco-burning products.[32]

The American Lung Association's "State of the Air" report in 2020 shows that too many cities across the nation increased the number of days when particle pollution, often called "soot," soared to often record-breaking levels. More cities suffered from higher numbers of days when ground-level ozone, also known as "smog," reached unhealthy levels. Many cities saw their year-round levels of particle pollution increase as well. The "State of the Air" report also adds to the evidence that a changing climate is making it harder to protect human health. The three years covered in this report ranked among the five hottest years on record globally. High ozone days and spikes in particle pollution followed, putting millions more people at risk and adding challenges to the work cities are doing across the nation to clean up the air. Nearly five in 10 people live where the air is unhealthy. 150 million Americans or approximately 45.8% of the population live in counties with unhealthy ozone or particle pollution. Los Angeles remains the city with the worst ozone pollution in the nation, as it has for 20 years of the 21-year history of the report. Bakersfield, CA, returned to the most polluted slot for year-round particle pollution, while Fresno-Madera-Hanford, CA, returned to its rank as the city with the worst short-term particle pollution. In contrast and for a breath of fresh air, some of the U.S. cities with the cleanest air are: Santa Fe, New Mexico, followed by Honolulu, Hawaii; Cheyenne, Wyoming; Great Falls, Montana; and Farmington, New Mexico.

One particular air pollution hub in the LA region is the 710 Freeway Corridor, also known as the diesel death yard. The region is made up of 20 neighborhoods that line Interstate 710. The area stretches from the ports of Los Angeles and Long Beach all the way up to central Los Angeles. The Ports of Long Beach and Los Angeles are the entry point of 40% of all imports to the U.S. and 20% of diesel particulate emissions in Southern California. Approximately 2,000 premature deaths are associated with diesel emissions in the corridor. Studies find that those living here are much more likely to develop asthma, heart disease, and lung cancer, and women are more likely to give birth prematurely.

To make matters even worse for the formerly Golden State, 2020 saw a series of wildfires that engulfed the state in smoke for several months. That smoke led to a 10% increase in asthma-related hospital admissions. As the impact of global warming continues, we will continue to see more extreme fires.[33]

As previously noted, air pollutants are ozone and particles, and both are largely products of cars and trucks. Research has demonstrated that these two substances contribute to heart disease, lung cancer, asthma attacks, and interfere with the growth and function of the lungs. Particle pollution is a combination of fine solids and aerosols that are suspended in the air we breathe.[34,35,36,37] Ozone is formed when nitrogen oxides (NOx) and hydrocarbons, or volatile organic compounds (VOCs) mix in the presence of sunlight:[38]

The Health Effects of Ozone

The effects of ozone on lung health have been studied at length using laboratory animals, clinical subjects and human populations. Two important studies released in late 2004 confirm that short-term exposure to ozone can kill. One study looked at 95 cities across the United States over a 14-year period. That study compared the impact of ozone on death patterns during several days after periods of relatively higher ozone levels. Even on days when ozone levels were below the current national standard, the researchers found an increased risk of premature death associated with increased levels of ozone. They estimated that over 3,700 deaths annually could be attributed to a 10 parts per billion increase in ozone levels.[39]

People can usually feel when ozone levels are high. Common symptoms include shortness of breath, chest pain when inhaling deeply, and eye irritation. Those who have asthma have a worsening of their condition when exposed to ozone.

Other Outdoor Air Pollutants

Carbon Monoxide (CO) is also a product of the burning of gasoline, natural gas, coal, and oil. It reduces the ability of blood to bring oxygen to body cells and tissues. Carbon monoxide may be particularly hazardous to people who have heart or circulatory (blood vessel) problems, and people who have damaged lungs or breathing passages. Sulfur dioxide is a product of the burning of coal and oil, especially high-sulfur coal from the Eastern United States and other industrial processes.[40] It may cause permanent damage to lungs, and also contributes to acid rain. And good old dust and smoke can also be significant air pollutants. Dust and smoke may irritate healthy people's eyes, nose, throat, and lungs, and might cause more serious problems in sensitive populations such as those with asthma and cardiovascular conditions.

Indoor Air Pollution

People spend the majority of their lives indoors: it is estimated that people spend around 90% of their life indoors.[41] While most indoor air is suitable and sometimes even better than outdoor air, there are many indoor air pollutants, and such pollutants end up being a significant source of illness and death in the U.S. especially when tobacco smoke is considered. Some indoor air pollutants are obvious (smoke in a room) but many are not visible and odorless and so many people are not aware that they are being exposed when they are being exposed. While much is known about indoor environment pollutants there are many things that are unknown; there is considerable uncertainty about what concentrations or periods of exposure to pollutants are necessary to produce specific health problems. Health effects from indoor air pollutants may be experienced soon after exposure or, possibly, years later. Short-term effects can include such things as irritation of the eyes, nose, and throat, headaches, dizziness, and fatigue. Exposure to some substances, like high levels of carbon monoxide, can cause immediate and serious illness. Reactions to indoor air pollutants depend on several factors like age and preexisting medical conditions. Those who have diseases like asthma, for example, might experience a worsening of their condition after exposure to indoor pollutants. In other cases, whether a person reacts to a pollutant depends on individual sensitivity, which varies tremendously from person to person. Some people can become sensitized to biological pollutants after repeated exposures, and it appears that some people can become sensitized to chemical pollutants as well. Other health problems (lung disease, heart diseases, cancer) may show up either years after exposure has occurred or only after long or repeated periods of exposure. Exposure to asbestos, for example, may lead to lung cancer 20 years after an exposure.

There are many sources of indoor air pollution. These include combustion sources such as oil, gas, kerosene, coal, wood, and tobacco products; building materials and furnishings, asbestos-containing insulation, wet or damp carpet, and furniture made of certain pressed wood products; products for household cleaning and maintenance, personal care, or hobbies; central heating and cooling systems and humidification devices; insects, and outdoor sources such as radon, pesticides, and other outdoor air pollutants.[42] The relative importance of any single source depends on how much of a given pollutant it emits and how hazardous those emissions are. Some sources, such as building materials, furnishings, and household products, like air fresheners, release pollutants more or less continuously. Other sources, related to activities carried out in the home like painting, using pesticides, and cleaning, release pollutants intermittently. Natural ventilation also affects the concentration of indoor air pollutants. If too little outdoor air enters buildings then pollutants can accumulate to levels that can pose health and comfort problems. Mechanical ventilation (HVAC systems) also influence pollutant levels and can sometimes add pollutants. Most people, especially those who inhabit office buildings and high rises, are largely dependent on mechanical ventilation. Humidity also affects pollutant levels and air quality. Elevated relative humidity at a surface can lead to problems with mold, corrosion, decay and other moisture-related deterioration.

When relative humidity reaches 100%, condensation can occur on surfaces leading to a whole host of additional problems. An elevated relative humidity in carpet and within fabrics can lead to dust mite infestation and mildew.[43] Outdoor air is another source of indoor air pollution. Sources of outdoor air pollution, such as power plants, can contribute to indoor air pollution. Outdoor air enters and leaves a building by infiltration; natural ventilation; and mechanical ventilation. Outdoor air can flow into a building through openings, joints, and cracks in walls, floors, and ceilings, and around windows and doors. In natural ventilation, air moves through opened windows and doors.[44]

Significant indoor air pollutants include radon, carbon monoxide, formaldehyde, volatile organic compounds, lead, tobacco smoke, pesticides, molds, asbestos, microbes, and insects. Radon is a known carcinogen and the EPA estimates that radon causes about 14,000 deaths per year in the United States. The most common source of indoor radon is uranium in the soil or rock on which homes are built. As uranium naturally breaks down, it releases radon gas which is a colorless, odorless, radioactive gas. Radon gas enters buildings through dirt floors, cracks in concrete walls and floors, floor drains, and sumps. Smoking greatly increases the risk of cancer from radon exposure.[45] Formaldehyde is another significant indoor air pollutant. Building materials including carpeting and plywood emit formaldehyde (H_2CO) gas. Formaldehyde is also used in numerous household products and is a by-product of combustion and certain other natural processes. Smoking is another source of formaldehyde. The rate at which products like pressed wood or textiles release formaldehyde varies; formaldehyde emissions generally decrease as products age. When products are new, high indoor temperatures or humidity can cause increased release of formaldehyde from these products. Formaldehyde, a colorless, pungent-smelling gas, can cause watery eyes, burning sensations in the eyes and throat, nausea, and difficulty in breathing in some humans exposed at elevated levels (above 0.1 parts per million). High concentrations may trigger attacks in people with asthma. Formaldehyde has also been shown to cause cancer in animals and may cause cancer in humans.[46] Organic chemicals (VOCs) are another source of indoor air pollution. Organic chemicals are widely used as ingredients in a variety of household products. Paints, varnishes, and wax all contain organic solvents, as do many cleaning, disinfecting, cosmetic, degreasing, and hobby products. Fuels are also made up of organic chemicals. The ability of these organic chemicals to cause health effects varies greatly, from those that are highly toxic, to those with no known health effect. As with other pollutants, the extent and nature of the health effect depends on many factors including level of exposure and length of time exposed. Eye and respiratory tract irritation, headaches, dizziness, visual disorders, and memory impairment are among the immediate symptoms that some people have experienced soon after exposure to some organic compounds. Many organic compounds are known to cause cancer in animals; some are suspected of causing, or are known to cause, cancer in humans.[47]

Carbon monoxide (CO) is a quick and silent killer, and it kills around 5,000 people per year. Lethal carbon monoxide poisoning is often caused by faulty vents and chimneys, or by the burning of charcoal indoors. Chronic carbon monoxide poisoning can result even from poorly adjusted pilot lights. Carbon monoxide (CO) is a colorless, odorless gas that interferes with the delivery of oxygen throughout the body. At high concentrations it can cause unconsciousness and death. Lower concentrations can cause a range of symptoms from headaches, dizziness, weakness, nausea, confusion, and disorientation, to fatigue in healthy people and episodes of increased chest pain in people with chronic heart disease. The symptoms of carbon monoxide poisoning are sometimes confused with the flu or food poisoning. Fetuses, infants, elderly people, and people with anemia or with a history of heart or respiratory disease can be especially sensitive to carbon monoxide exposures.[48] Nitrogen dioxide (NO_2) is another product of combustion that causes indoor air pollution. Nitrogen dioxide is a colorless, odorless gas that irritates the mucous membranes in the eye, nose, and throat, and causes shortness of breath after exposure to high concentrations. There is evidence that high concentrations or continued exposure to low levels of nitrogen dioxide increases the risk of respiratory infection; there is also evidence from animal studies that repeated exposures to elevated nitrogen dioxide levels may lead, or contribute, to the development of emphysema. People at particular risk from exposure to nitrogen dioxide include children and individuals with asthma and other respiratory diseases.[49]

Perchloroethylene, a chemical most widely used in dry cleaning, is another source of indoor air pollution, and it has been shown to cause cancer in animals and is suspected of causing cancer in humans. Recent studies indicate that people breathe low levels of perchloroethylene both in homes where dry-cleaned goods are stored and as they wear dry-cleaned clothing.[50]

Lead is another pollutant of concern and is fairly common in the urban environment, especially in older buildings. Lead paint can degenerate into dust and be inhaled. Lead has long been recognized as a harmful environmental pollutant. In late 1991, the Secretary of the Department of Health and Human Services called lead the number one environmental threat to the health of children in the United States. There are many ways in which humans are exposed to lead: through air, drinking water, food, contaminated soil, deteriorating paint, and dust. Airborne lead enters the body when an individual breathes or swallows lead particles or dust once it has settled. Before it was known how harmful lead could be, lead was used in paint, gasoline, water pipes, and many other products. Old lead-based paint is the most significant source of lead exposure in the U.S. today. Harmful exposures to lead can be created when lead-based paint is improperly removed from surfaces by dry scraping, sanding, or open-flame burning. High concentrations of airborne lead particles in homes can also result from lead dust from outdoor sources, including contaminated soil tracked inside, and use of lead in certain indoor activities such as soldering and stained-glass making. Lead affects practically all systems within the body. At high levels it can cause convulsions, coma, and even death. Lower levels of lead can adversely affect the brain, central nervous system, blood cells, and kidneys. The effects of lead exposure on fetuses and young children can be severe. Such effects include delays in physical and mental development, lower IQ levels, shortened attention spans, and increased behavioral problems.[51]

One particular East LA neighborhood became the poster for lead contamination concerns when it was discovered that a battery manufacturer, Exide, had basically polluted the entire neighborhood with lead. Since the 1970s, Exide had been blanketing the neighborhood with lead and other heavy metals. In 2013, the Air Quality Management District explained that upwards of 250,000 residents in East Los Angeles face a chronic health hazard from lead and arsenic exposure from Exide. Communities living near Exide such as Boyle Heights and Maywood are more than 90% Latino and rank among the top 10% of most environmentally burdened areas in California. More than 90% of homes in the area were built before the 1978 ban on lead paint and many directly neighbor freeways and truck routes which resulted in decades of exposure to leaded gasoline which contaminated soil. Lead exposure is especially prevalent in soil, water, and dust there. In 2019, a study conducted by the University of Southern California found a high amount of lead in baby teeth of children in Boyle Heights, Maywood, East Los

Angeles, Commerce, and Huntington Park. The lead in the baby teeth matched with soil contamination data from the California Department of Toxic Substances Control. The Truth Fairy study revealed that children in Boyle Heights and East LA have the highest exposure to lead, which most likely came through winds carrying soil in utero from their mother or post birth.[52]

Pesticides are another significant indoor air pollutant. Around 75% of U.S. households used at least one pesticide product indoors per year. Products used most often are insecticides and disinfectants. Pesticides used in and around the home include products to control insects (insecticides), termites (termiticides), rodents (rodenticides), fungi (fungicides), and microbes (disinfectants). The health effects of pesticide exposures range from irritation to eye, nose, and throat; damage to central nervous system and kidney; and increased risk of cancer.[53]

Relatedly, cockroaches and other insects end up being a significant source of indoor air pollution. For those who have lived in older buildings in the big city, you know that many buildings are simply infested with cockroaches. No, cockroaches don't crawl in your lungs, but their saliva, feces and shedding body parts can trigger both asthma and allergies. These allergens act like dust mites, aggravating symptoms when they are kicked up in the air. The National Pest Management Association reports that 63% of homes in the United States contain cockroach allergens. In urban areas, that number rises to between 78% and 98% of homes.

Asbestos, a mineral fiber that has been used in the past for insulation and as a fire-retardant, is known to cause lung disease (asbestosis) and lung cancer, and is another known indoor air pollutant. Today, asbestos is most commonly found in older homes, in pipe and furnace insulation materials, asbestos shingles, millboard, textured paints and other coating materials, and floor tiles. Elevated concentrations of airborne asbestos can occur after asbestos-containing materials are disturbed by cutting, sanding or other remodeling activities. Improper attempts to remove these materials can release asbestos fibers into the air. After the asbestos fibers are inhaled, they can remain and accumulate in the lungs. Most people with asbestos-related diseases were exposed to elevated concentrations on the job; some developed disease from exposure to clothing and equipment brought home from job sites. Smokers are at higher risk of developing asbestos-induced lung cancer.[54]

Biological sources of air pollution can also be found indoors, and they include bacteria, molds, mildew, viruses, animal dander and cat saliva, house dust mites, cockroaches, and pollen. There are many sources of these pollutants. Pollens originate from plants; viruses are transmitted by people and animals; bacteria are carried by people, animals, and soil and plant debris; and household pets are sources of saliva and animal dander. The protein in urine from rats and mice is a potent allergen. When it dries, it can become airborne. Contaminated central air handling systems can become breeding grounds for mold, mildew, and other sources of biological contaminants, and can then distribute these contaminants through the home. There are several factors that influence the levels of biological pollutants in the indoor environment including humidity, temperature and presence of standing water. House dust mites, one of the most powerful biological allergens, grow in damp, warm environments. Biological contaminants can trigger allergic reactions, including hypersensitivity pneumonitis, allergic rhinitis, and some types of asthma. Allergic reactions occur only after repeated exposure to a specific biological allergen. However, a reaction may occur immediately upon re-exposure or after multiple exposures over time. As a result, people who have noticed only mild allergic reactions, or no reactions at all, may suddenly find themselves very sensitive to particular allergens.[55]

While there are many identified indoor air pollutants, there are occasions where no particular agents can be identified yet the people who occupy a building feel sick. The term "sick building syndrome" (SBS) is used to describe situations in which building occupants experience acute health and comfort effects that appear to be linked to time spent in a building, but no specific illness or cause can be identified. The complaints may be localized in a particular room or zone, or may be widespread throughout the building. Symptoms of SBS illness include: headache; eye, nose, or throat irritation; dry cough; dry or itchy skin; dizziness and nausea; difficulty in concentrating; fatigue; and sensitivity to odors. Inadequate ventilation is often at the heart of SBS. Other culprits are thought to be indoor and outdoor chemical contaminants, and biological contaminants. Legionnaires' disease is caused by a bacterium that is peculiar to HVAC systems and the bug was only discovered after many people got "sick" in a building.[56]

Can You Drink the Water?

We never know the worth of water till the well is dry.
~ Thomas Fuller

Water is essential for life, and access to a safe water supply along with adequate sanitation are essential for a community to function. Adults require between two and three quarts of water per day; a person can only live for five to seven days without water. Some 1.7 million deaths a year worldwide are attributable to unsafe water and to poor sanitation. Most of the deaths occur in children, and virtually all occur in developing countries.[57] Most city dwellers depend on municipal suppliers for their water needs. U.S. drinking water is, of course, treated and highly regulated. The quality of drinking water has clearly improved over time; thousands of city dwellers died in the past because of contaminated drinking water. In the seventeenth century, the invention of the microscope by Anton van Leeuwenhoek and his discovery of microorganisms, and the design of the multiple filter by Luca Antonio Porzio helped lead to an understanding of the role of microbes in waterborne illness and how water could be treated. During the mid to late 1800s, scientists gained a greater understanding of the sources and effects of drinking water contaminants, especially those that were not visible to the naked eye. In 1855, epidemiologist Dr. John Snow proved that cholera was a waterborne disease by linking an outbreak of illness in London to a public well that was contaminated by sewage. In the 1870s, Dr. Robert Koch and Dr. Joseph Lister demonstrated that microorganisms existing in water supplies cause disease. The first water facility to deliver water to an entire town was built in Paisley, Scotland in 1804 by John Gibb and was used to supply his bleachery and the town. Within three years this filtered water was piped directly to customers in Glasgow, Scotland.[58] America has relied on several processes of water treatment to progressively ensure the water quality. Early treatment was mostly done by filtration, but because distribution systems were extended to serve a growing population – as people have moved from concentrated urban areas to more suburban areas – additional disinfection was instituted to keep water safe. Today, filtration and chlorination are the standard treatments used to protect U.S. water supplies from harmful microbes. In the 1970s and 1980s, improvements were made in membrane development for reverse osmosis filtration and other treatment techniques such as ozonation. Some treatment advancements have been driven by the discovery of chlorine-resistant pathogens in drinking water that can cause illnesses like hepatitis and cryptosporidiosis. Other advancements have resulted from the need to remove more and more chemicals found in sources of drinking water.[59] At present most municipalities still use chlorine to disinfect water. Almost all of the remaining surface water systems, and some of the remaining groundwater systems, use other disinfectants, such as ozone or chloramine to treat water. And while there have been substantial improvements in the provision of safe drinking water in the U.S. since the enactment of the Clean Water Act, the Safe Drinking Water Act and the National Secondary Drinking Water Regulations, many people are still unsure if it is safe to "drink the water" and they should be. The National Resources Defense Council (NRDC) monitors the nation's drinking water, and have found that pollution and deteriorating and out-of-date plumbing are delivering drinking water that poses health risks to some residents. The rather old-fashioned water treatment that most municipalities use to filter out particles in the water and kill some parasites and bacteria generally fails to remove 21st-century contaminants like pesticides, industrial chemicals and arsenic. A NRDC report found confirmed violations of enforceable tap water rules in many cities. Milwaukee, Pittsburgh, Detroit and, of course, Flint, topped the list. In 2018, 57 of Detroit's public schools tested positive for surplus amounts of lead, which led to a temporary shutoff of water fountains, and new filtration systems were added in said schools citywide. Aside from poor water quality, from 2014-2017, more than 100,000 families in Detroit had their water shut off because they couldn't afford the bills – insult to injury. In 2014, officials failed to apply corrosion inhibitors to Flint's water when it changed sources from the Detroit Water and Sewage Department to the Flint River. As a result, thousands of people were exposed to extremely dangerous levels of lead and bacteria. Officially, 90 people fell ill and 12 died. However, a later investigation found that 115 residents died from pneumonia at the time which actually could've been caused by waterborne bacteria in the area. Rural water has its issues too, less than most municipalities, but the difference is that you might, as an individual, have the power to help fix it.

Another drinking water concern is what happens to the water after it leaves the city's pipes and enters residential plumbing.

Those living in older buildings are at risk of being exposed to lead that generally occurs from the corrosion of lead pipes either between the water main and the tap. A lot of urbanites don't drink tap water and drink bottled water instead, but bottled water sold in the U.S. is not necessarily cleaner or safer than most tap water, according to a four-year scientific study by NRDC. There has been an explosion in bottled water use in the United States over the past 20 years driven in large measure by marketing designed to convince the public of bottled water's purity and safety, and capitalizing on public concern about tap water quality. The NRDC did a study of more than 1,000 bottles of 103 brands of bottled water. While most of the tested waters were found to be of high quality, some brands were contaminated: about one-third of the waters tested contained levels of contamination including synthetic organic chemicals, bacteria, and arsenic. A key finding of the study was that bottled water regulations are inadequate to assure consumers of either purity or safety, although both the federal government and the states have bottled water safety programs. At the national level, the Food and Drug Administration (FDA) is responsible for bottled water safety, but the FDA's rules completely exempt waters that are packaged and sold within the same state, which account for between 60 and 70 percent of all bottled water sold in the United States (roughly one out of five states don't regulate these waters either). The FDA also exempts carbonated water and seltzer, and fewer than half of the states require carbonated waters to meet their own bottled water standards. Even when bottled waters are covered by the FDA's rules, they are subject to less rigorous testing and purity standards than those which apply to city tap water. For example, bottled water is required to be tested less frequently than city tap water for bacteria and chemical contaminants. In addition, bottled water rules allow for some contamination by E. coli or fecal coliform (which indicate possible contamination with fecal matter), contrary to tap water rules, which prohibit any confirmed contamination with these bacteria. Similarly, there are no requirements for bottled water to be disinfected or tested for parasites such as cryptosporidium or giardia, unlike the rules for big city tap water systems that use surface water sources. Some bottled water then may present a health threat to people with weakened immune systems, such as the frail elderly, some infants, transplant or cancer patients, or people with HIV/AIDS.[60] And yes, whatever those bottles are made of, make their way into the water and into you. Lastly, bottled water is often actually just tap water. Know where your bottled water is sourced from before you drink it.

Natural Disasters in the Unnatural World

There's no disaster that can't become a blessing, and no blessing that can't become a disaster.
~ Richard Bach

Even though city dwellers live in a largely unnatural world, every so often the natural world does something to remind urbanites that they live on planet earth. Over the past five years the world has experienced a number of devastating calamities including the 2004 Indian Ocean tsunami which killed over 200,000 people and the Hurricane Katrina disaster. There are many weather-related and geological phenomena ranging from inclement weather to earthquakes that can impact the lives of city dwellers. Hurricane Katrina (2005) was the costliest and one of the deadliest hurricanes in the history of the United States. It was the sixth-strongest Atlantic hurricane ever recorded and the third-strongest landfalling U.S. hurricane. Katrina formed in late August during the 2005 Atlantic hurricane season and devastated much of the north-central Gulf Coast of the United States. Levees separating Lake Pontchartrain from New Orleans were breached by the storm surge, ultimately flooding 80% of the city and many areas of neighboring parishes for weeks. Katrina is estimated to be responsible for $81.2 billion in damages, making it the costliest natural disaster in U.S. history. The storm killed at least 1,836 people, making it the deadliest U.S. hurricane.[61] The city of New Orleans lost more than half of its population due to Hurricane Katrina. Since Katrina, there have been many other hurricanes...

Los Angeles and San Francisco are well known for their earthquakes, but earthquakes can occur almost anywhere in the U.S. The Loma Prieta earthquake in San Francisco in 1989 registered 6.9 on the Richter scale, and killed 63 people and caused massive damage. The last major quake to hit L.A., the Northridge earthquake, which occurred on January 17, 1994, registered 6.7 magnitude on the Richter scale and killed approximately 50 people and injured over 9,000. Of the 50 who died, it appears that 20 died as a result of a heart attack.[62] The Kobe (population 1.5 million) earthquake in Japan which followed a year later also demonstrated how damaging and deadly earthquakes can be in urban settings. The earthquake was the most damaging to strike Japan since the great Kanto earthquake destroyed large areas of Tokyo and Yokohama and killed 143,000 people in 1923. The Kobe quake killed 5,096 people and injured 26,797. One-fifth of the city's population was left homeless, and more than 103,521 buildings were destroyed. Most of the deaths and injuries occurred when older wood-frame houses with heavy clay tile roofs collapsed. The collapse of these buildings was followed by the ignition of over 300 fires within minutes of the earthquake. Response to the fires was hindered by the failure of the water supply system and the disruption of the traffic system.[63]

Extremes of heat and cold can also impact urbanites. Many urbanites die every year from heat-related illness, and it appears that heat will kill more in the future as the earth continues to heat up. Urban environments are unique for their heat island effect – urban environs typically run between 2 to 10°F (1 to 6°C) hotter than surrounding rural areas. Heat-related illnesses (e.g., heat cramps, heat exhaustion, heat syncope, or heatstroke) can occur when high ambient temperatures overcome the body's natural ability to dissipate heat. Older adults, young children, and persons with chronic medical conditions are particularly susceptible to these illnesses and are at high risk for heat-related mortality. Across the country, heat caused at least 10,000 deaths between 1999 and 2016 – more than hurricanes, tornadoes or floods in most years.

Scientists link the warming planet to a rise in dangerous heat in the U.S., as well as the spread of infectious diseases and other health conditions. Federal research predicts heatstroke and similar illnesses will claim tens of thousands of American lives each year by the end of the century. Already, higher temperatures pose lethal risks: the five warmest years nationwide have all occurred since 2006. In the last six decades, the number of annual heat waves in 50 U.S. cities has, on average, tripled. The states with the highest average annual hyperthermia-related death rate are Arizona, followed by Nevada and Missouri. The 1995 Chicago heat wave led to approximately 600 heat-related deaths over a period of five days. It is now considered to be one of the worst weather-related disasters in American history.[64]

Cold weather can also kill people, though most hypothermia deaths occur in non-urban environments. Hypothermia, a lowering of the core body temperature to <95° F (<35° C), causes approximately 600 deaths each year in the United States. Alcohol plays a major role in many hypothermia deaths. Certain populations (e.g., alcoholics; drug users; elderly, homeless, and chronically ill persons; and those with preexisting heart disease) are at increased risk for dying from hypothermia.

Ultraviolet radiation is another environmental agent that harms and kills urbanites. Ultraviolet (UV) rays are a part of sunlight, and the rays can penetrate and change the structure of skin cells. There are three types of UV rays: ultraviolet A (UVA), ultraviolet B (UVB), and ultraviolet C (UVC). UVA is the most abundant source of solar radiation at the earth's surface and penetrates beyond the top layer of human skin. Scientists believe that UVA radiation can cause damage to connective tissue and increase a person's risk for developing skin cancer. UVB rays are less abundant at the earth's surface than UVA because a significant portion of UVB rays is absorbed by the ozone layer. Unfortunately, because of a massive hole in the ozone layer, more UVB rays are getting in. UVB rays penetrate less deeply into the skin than do UVA rays, but also can be damaging. One in five Americans will develop skin cancer in their lifetime, and one American dies every hour from the disease. Melanoma, the most serious form of skin cancer, is also one of the fastest growing types of cancer in the United States. Melanoma cases in this country have more than doubled in the past two decades, and the rise is expected to continue. Nonmelanoma skin cancers are less deadly than melanomas, but they can spread and further hurt and kill people. More than 1.2 million Americans develop nonmelanoma skin cancer a year and around 1,900 die from the disease. Damaging UV rays are more common at higher elevations and in the South and West.

Chapter 4

Bodily Harm

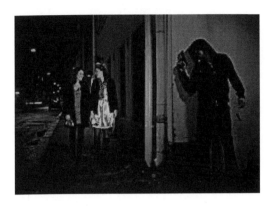

One who is injured ought not to return the injury, for on no account can it be right to do an injustice; and it is not right to return an injury, or to do evil to any man, however much we have suffered from him.

~ Socrates

Bodily harm is injury. Injury is defined as physical damage to an individual that occurs over a short period of time as a result of acute exposure. The major categories of injury are intentional, unintentional, and occupational. Intentional injuries result from interpersonal or self-inflicted violence, and include homicide, assaults, suicide and suicide attempts, child abuse and neglect, intimate partner violence, elder abuse, and sexual assault. Unintentional injuries are injuries that result from motor vehicle collisions, falls, fires, poisonings, and drownings.

When one thinks "city" one often thinks "danger." Violence seems to be deeply rooted in American society and has become a fixture in most city dweller's lives. When measured against comparable industrialized nations, America is indeed a violent country and a good chunk of the violence in America occurs in big cities. While U.S. cities aren't the most violent cities in the world, the homicide rates of our most violent cities are much higher than those of other industrialized countries. A study from the Harvard School of Public Health, for example, found that among high income nations, the United States has the highest rate of female homicide victimization, and they concluded that our high rate of homicide is tied to our high rate of gun ownership. Among those ages 15 to 24, the U.S. firearm homicide rate is five times higher than in neighboring Canada and 30 times higher than in Japan.[65] There has been a dramatic increase in deaths caused by violent acts during the past one hundred years in the U.S. In 1900 the homicide rate was approximately 1 per 100,000 people and by 1990 it reached 10 per 100,000.[66] Gangs are now omnipresent in all big cities. And in addition to the homegrown violence Americans now face international threats as well: the terrorist attacks of 9/11 killed approximately 3,000 people. Other bodily harm concerns for urbanites include transportation, work, and home-related incidents and accidents. While big cities per se are often not the location of our all too common mass shootings – Aurora, Sandy Hook – it takes little imagination to realize that any area where masses of people are gathered are potential targets for such events. It's just a question of time before some disturbed soul decides to open up on a crowd of people in one of our big cities.

The city can be a dangerous place to live, but one's risk of harm is related to a variety of factors: income, ethnicity, access to firearms, gender, occupation, neighborhood, education, mental health status, community involvement, police presence, and the use of drugs and alcohol.

When a person gets injured their physical injury can also negatively impact their mental health and other facets of their life. Victims of rape, for example, often experience chronic headaches, fatigue, sleep disturbances, recurrent nausea, decreased appetite, eating disorders, menstrual pain, sexual dysfunction, and suicidal behavior.[67] It is also important to note that injuries affect more than just the injured person. With a nonfatal injury, family members are often called upon to care for the injured person, which can result in stress, time away from work, and possibly lost income. With a fatal injury, family, friends, coworkers, employers, and other members of the injured person's community feel the loss. When someone gets injured it becomes everyone's problem. When someone gets murdered it's everyone's loss. Injuries are a major public health issue; they cause a lot of deaths and disability, especially in urban settings.

United States Injury Facts

Thousands of Americans are killed and hurt each year as a result of injury. People get murdered, raped, shot, and assaulted in the U.S. every day. People fall, drown, and get burned. People crash their cars, trains derail, and planes fall from the sky. And people commit suicide. While most Americans die from heart disease and cancer, the amount of injury death in the U.S. is substantial. Most of those impacted by injury, especially violent injury, are young. Alcohol is a major contributor to bodily harm in the U.S. – intoxicated people tend to crash cars and fight. In some communities, especially the inner city, violent injury is at epidemic levels. Homicide is the second leading cause of death for Americans ages 15 to 34. Unintentional injuries are the leading cause of death for those under 35 years of age. And while thousands of people are murdered in the U.S. each year, usually twice as many commit suicide. Suicide is the second highest ranked cause of death for those between 25 and 34 years of age, and the third most frequent for those between 10 and 24. Other facts:

- In the United States, more than seven people per hour die a violent death. More than 19,500 people were victims of homicide and over 47,000 people died by suicide in 2017 alone.

- Excessive alcohol consumption is an important factor in more than 100,000 injury deaths in the U.S. each year.

- Males have higher injury risks than females as males are more likely than females to engage in behaviors that put them at risk. Males are at least four times as likely as women to die from suicide.

- Over 700,000 rapes occur each year. Only 16% of rape victims report the offense to police. 25% of women reported being raped or physically assaulted by an intimate partner at some time in their lives. Most physical and sexual assaults are perpetrated by known assailants.

- More than half of those killed in motor vehicle accidents were not wearing seatbelts.

- Most murders and rapes occur in July.

- Most poisoning deaths are caused by pills, alcohols, gases and fumes, and chemicals.

- Most murders occur in conjunction with another crime, especially robbery, and many occur in association with an argument (44%). Most murders are committed by known assailants.

- Per mile driven, adults 65 and older have a higher crash rate than all but teen drivers, and the pedestrian death rate for people 65 and older is higher than for any other age group. Falls are the leading cause of injury-related death among this age group.

- Older adults are among those at greatest risk for injuries from residential fires. Older adults have the highest suicide rate.

- 2.8 million people were hospitalized due to injuries in 2015.

- 27.6 million people were treated in an emergency department for injuries in 2015.

- Motor vehicle crashes are a leading cause of injury death in the U.S. More than 35,000 people died from motor vehicle crashes in 2015.

- Opioid overdoses have quadrupled since 1999, with more than 15,000 people dying from prescription opioid overdoses in 2015.

Intentional Injury

Violent crime is a major concern for city dwellers. Everyday there are news reports of drive-by shootings, carjackings, home invasion robberies, serial rapists and the like in big cities in the U.S. Most large cities have those fear-provoking neighborhoods; places that are scary during the day and even scarier at night. And in addition to the usual property-related assaults and assaults where the assailant is known to the victim, cities have also spawned a fair number of serial killers, e.g., Charles Manson, Son of Sam, the Zodiac Killer, and the Green River Killer.

The reputation of big cities as violent is fairly well entrenched and the reputation, for the most part, is fairly well deserved, especially in poorer "inner-city" neighborhoods. While violent crime had taken a bit of a dip during the past 10 years until 2020 hit, statistics continue to demonstrate that big cities are typically more violent than other communities. Department of Justice statistics reveal that the largest cities (those with 250,000 and over in population) experienced the highest murder rate among the city population groups (12.5 murders per 100,000 inhabitants). The smallest cities (those under 10,000 in population) had the lowest murder rate (2.4 offenses per 100,000 inhabitants). Big cities also had higher rape rates.[68] Several organizations rank cities based on murder and violent crime rates. In 2019, FBI data show there were an estimated 366.7 violent crimes per 100,000 residents in the United States. Surprisingly, Anchorage, Alaska is the new per capita murder capital of the United States. Albuquerque and Memphis weren't far behind. On the other side, Provo, Lancaster and Portland were among the lowest. Anchorage is dangerous, you ask? That's drugs, alcohol and too many males.

Gang members are responsible for a lot of urban murders. It is estimated that nearly half of murders in Los Angeles and Chicago are gang related. Around 800,000 gang members and 25,000 gangs were active in more than 2,900 jurisdictions in the U.S. Los Angeles is well known for its gangs and some LA gangs have spread across the U.S. and to other countries. In Los Angeles County, law enforcement officials estimate that there are more than 1,300 street gangs with over 150,000 members. In the City of Los Angeles alone, there are approximately 407 gangs and over 56,000 members. The Crips are one of LA's biggest gangs. The Crips got their start in the late 1960s and usually identify with the color blue in several different shades often wearing a blue rag or handkerchief as an identity item. The Bloods, another infamous LA gang, began as the Piru Street Gang in the seventies and they typically wear red. The Crips and Bloods have historically been fierce rivals and have been responsible for a lot of murders in LA... and they're still around. The Mara Salvatrucha gang (also known as MS-13), which also started in LA, was formed by immigrants from El Salvador in the eighties. Various members of the original gang got arrested and deported back to El Salvador and the gang flourished there and spread through Central America and continues to grow in the U.S. The gang has a uniquely international profile, with an estimated 8,000 to 10,000 members in 33 states in the United States, and tens of thousands more in Central America. It's considered the fastest-growing, most violent street gang.

While some big U.S. cities have higher violent crime rates than other living environments, it is not exactly clear why they do. As Steven Levitt pointed out in *Freakonomics*, it is unclear even to crime experts what makes violent crime rates rise and fall; violent crime is not a simple matter.[69] Violent crimes appear to be associated with degree of urbanization; percentage of youth in the population; stability of population; modes of transportation; economic conditions, especially inequality; cultural, education, and religious factors; lack of recreational opportunities; family conditions; climate; urban blight; quality of law enforcement; availability of weapons; and strength of community bonding and trust. Many of the above-noted factors are part of the urban landscape. While many city dwellers fear that they will be murdered by some unknown assailant as they innocently walk down the street, violent acts are more common between people who know each other. Homicide victims and assailants traditionally have been more likely to be acquainted and share the same race. Most victims and assailants are male. Rape victims also typically know their assailants. Frequently, homicides begin with arguments; more often than not, they involve alcohol and firearms. Many, including the American Psychological Association (APA), have concluded that violence is learned behavior.[70] The belief is that young people – the group that accounts for most of the violence in the U.S. – are exposed to violence at home, in their neighborhood, and in the media, and decide to give violent behavior a shot. If the violent behavior works then they continue using violence to work their way through life. Big cities often have many of the requisite ingredients that contribute to violent behavior, but what makes one city more violent than another is not scientifically clear and some have argued that big cities really aren't that much more violent than other living environs. In *Murder in New York City*, Eric H. Monkkonen analyzed the changes in homicide rates in New York City over the past two hundred years. While cities, like New York City, are often thought of as cauldrons of murder, Monkkonen points out that for the first half of the twentieth century New York's homicide rate was lower than the rate for the U.S. as a whole. He also noted that New York's homicide rate increased as the city became less crowded; poverty and economic downturns were not associated with higher homicide rates; and that periods of high levels of police corruption and lack of public trust of police did not lead to more murders.[71] New York continues to have murder rates that are typically lower than the national average.

High population density is one feature that distinguishes urban communities from other communities and many have concluded that it is this high population density that leads to social disorder and violent crime. While this seems kind of logical there is little proof of such an association. There are many bigger and denser cities in other countries (e.g., Tokyo, London) that have much lower violent crime rates than U.S. cities. A lot of the "crowded cities make people violent" idea stems from J.B. Calhoun's 1962 study of rats in crowded conditions in which Calhoun demonstrated that rats began engaging in aberrant behavior (abnormal sexual patterns, cannibalism, hyperaggression) as the population became more dense. Sociologists and others then took Calhoun's study and concluded that it was this urban crowding that accounted for the human misbehavior (rape, murder, drug use); put people in crowded conditions and they'll attack each other.[72] Franz De Waal, Professor of Primate Behavior at Emory University and the Director of Living Links, Yerkes Primate Center, has studied primate behavior under a variety of conditions and does not believe that crowding alone accounts for high violent crime rates seen in some big cities. He feels that it is the combination of crowding, anonymity, weapon availability, and resource competition that leads to violent crime.[73]

From De Waal's "Coping with Crowding" (*Scientific American*):[74]

In no time, popularizers were comparing politically motivated street riots to rat packs, inner cities to behavioral sinks and urban areas to zoos warning that society was heading for either anarchy or dictatorship..

Robert Ardrey, an American science journalist, remarked in 1970 on the voluntary nature of human crowding:

Just as Calhoun's rats freely chose to eat in the middle pens, we freely enter the city. Calhoun's views soon became a central tenet of the voluminous literature on aggression. In extrapolating from rodents to people, however, these thinkers and writers were making a gigantic leap of faith. A look at human populations suggests why such a simple extrapolation is so problematic. Compare, for instance, per capita murder rates with the number of people per square kilometer in different nations – as we did, using data from the United Nations' 1996 Demographic Yearbook. If things were straightforward, the two ought to vary in tandem. Instead there is no statistically meaningful relation.

If there is something about cities that influences violent behavior then a significant part of that "something" appears to be the quality of the social environment. Robert Sampson, Professor of Sociology at Harvard, studied violent crime in Chicago and found that violent crime tends to cluster in certain neighborhoods, and in those same neighborhoods you often find high injury, infant mortality, and low birth weight rates. Health-related problems including injury are strongly associated with the social characteristics of communities and neighborhoods. Sampson studied 8,782 residents across several Chicago neighborhoods and found that in neighborhoods where collective efficacy was high – neighbors could be counted on to do things for the neighborhood – there were significantly lower rates of violence, as measured by official homicide events or as violent victimization reported by residents, even adjusting for prior neighborhood violence that may have depressed collective efficacy (e.g., because of fear). Overall, one standard deviation elevation in collective efficacy was associated with about a

13% reduction in the expected homicide rate.[75] The *Moving to Opportunity* (MTO) program was a HUD-based series of housing experiments that took place in five U.S. cities where housing project residents were randomly assigned to one of three groups: an experimental group that received housing subsidies to move into low-poverty (more affluent) neighborhoods; a group that received conventional (Section 8) housing assistance; and a control group that received no special assistance. A study from the Boston MTO site showed that children of mothers in the experimental group (those who moved to a more affluent neighborhood) had significantly lower prevalence of injuries, asthma attacks, and personal victimization during follow-up. The move to wealthier neighborhoods was also linked to lower violent offending among juveniles and to significant improvements in the general health status and mental health of household heads.[76] Lederman and Loayza's research for the World Bank showed that the sense of trust among community members had a significant negative effect on homicide rates as did lower rates of income disparity.[77] Margaret Zahn, a North Carolina State University criminologist and former President of the American Society of Criminology, has shown in her work that violent crime is tied to poverty.[78] Urban violent crime then, which for the most part takes place in the inner city, is influenced by social conditions including disparities of income, education, and opportunity; access to firearms; drugs and alcohol; policing; and learned violence. It is also possible that the anonymity factor of the big city (a lack of social connection and neighborhood involvement) is also a component of the high violent crime rates found in some of America's big cities.

Suicide

While suicide is clearly influenced by mental illness it is categorized as an intentional injury. Although urban suicide rates in the U.S. are not higher than suburban and rural rates, suicide accounts for many urban deaths every year. There are more suicide deaths each year than homicide deaths. More males commit suicide than females by a ratio of four to one and most are white. Young people (suicide is the third leading cause of death for those between 15 and 24 years of age) and older people are responsible for most suicide deaths in the U.S. Firearms are responsible for the majority of suicides.[79] Emile Durkheim, a 19th century French sociologist, believed that high suicide rates were associated with low levels of social integration. Durkheim defined social integration as being attached to social groups, maintaining interpersonal ties, and feeling allegiance to social groups. Low levels or an absence of social integration, as measured by living alone or experiencing marital disruption, represent social isolation and the atomization of individuals in a community.[80] Currently identified risk factors for suicide are:[81]

- Mental disorders, particularly mood disorders, schizophrenia, anxiety disorders and certain personality disorders
- Alcohol and other substance use disorders
- Hopelessness
- Impulsive and/or aggressive tendencies
- History of trauma or abuse
- Physical illnesses
- Previous suicide attempt
- Family history of suicide
- Job or financial loss
- Relational or social loss
- Easy access to lethal means
- Local clusters of suicide that have a contagious influence
- Lack of social support and sense of isolation
- Stigma associated with help-seeking behavior
- Barriers to accessing healthcare, especially mental health and substance abuse treatment

- Certain cultural and religious beliefs (for instance, the belief that suicide is a noble resolution of a personal dilemma)
- Exposure to, including through the media, and influence of others who have died by suicide

Other Sources of Urban Injury

Motor Vehicles

While many urbanites are concerned about violent crime, motor vehicles cause more deaths and injuries than violent crime. In 2003, there were 3,189,000 traffic injuries stemming from 2,070,000 injury crashes, compared with 910,774 aggravated assaults, a more than 3-to-1 ratio.[82] In 2016 total transportation fatalities were 39,565. Motor vehicle-related deaths make up a significant proportion of work-related deaths. And drinking while under the influence and not using seatbelts contribute to a significant proportion of automobile-related deaths in the U.S. While there are a higher percentage of fatal crashes in rural areas, there are still plenty of urban transportation-related deaths. Most transportation deaths occur on highways. As noted by William Lucy ("Mortality Risk Associated With Leaving Home: Recognizing the Relevance of the Built Environment"), the exurbs (beyond the suburbs) are the most dangerous region of metropolitan areas – cars move faster on two lane roads where dangers of driver impairment, mistakes, and inattention lead to accidents. Divided roads in general are much safer than undivided roads. Risk of fatal accidents is generally associated with speed. Typically only 10% of fatal accidents occur in speed zones of 30 miles per hour or less, compared with the 50% of fatalities that occur in speed zones of 55 miles per hour or more. Research has confirmed that people who drive farther each day (long-distance commuters), also drive faster. A study of effects of low-density suburban sprawl in 83 metropolitan areas found that traffic fatality rates were 50% higher in the 10 most sprawling than in the 10 least sprawling metropolitan areas – a rate of 36 fatalities, compared with 23, per 100,000 residents.[83] According to Lucy, long-distance commuting may actually be more dangerous than living in a violent inner city neighborhood; people fear bad neighborhoods, but they don't fear the highway. And while other forms of transportation are often safer than cars, some people are still killed each year via these other means of transportation, but it is dramatically lower per mile than automobile transportation.

While most people are civil and skilled drivers, there are plenty of drivers who aren't. Road rage is another motor vehicle-related bodily harm concern in metropolitan areas. There are millions of urban commuters, and commuting times are going up undoubtedly making commuters more frustrated. According to an Automobile Association of America (AAA) sponsored report on aggressive driving, an average of at least 1,500 men, women, and children are injured or killed each year in the United States as a result of "aggressive driving." While drivers are typically young, "roadragers" can be any age. Many aggressive drivers are relatively poorly educated males who have criminal records, histories of violence, and drug or alcohol problems. Many have recently suffered an emotional or professional setback, such as losing a job or a girlfriend, are going through a divorce, or have suffered an injury or an accident.[84] But many aggressive drivers – motorists who have snapped and committed vehicular violence – are successful men and women with no known histories of crime, violence, or alcohol and drug abuse. Anyone is capable of "going off" and wreaking havoc with their car. As noted in the study, Oscar-winner Jack Nicholson, for example, in 1994, believed that the driver of another car cut him off in traffic and he grabbed a golf club, stepped out of his car at a red light, and repeatedly struck the windshield and roof of the other driver's car. The AAA Foundation study revealed that one of the main factors influencing driver behavior was mood. It was suggested that this may be due to the fact that, for many of the unsafe drivers, the act of car driving is regarded as an expressive, rather than practical, activity. Being in a bad mood appears to have an adverse effect on driving behavior. Individuals vary enormously in their propensity to display aggression based on their experiences. The positive responses which previous expressions of aggression have elicited lead certain people to rely on aggressive behavior as a method to achieve their own ends. Driver aggression often reflects the level of aggression in the society. Whitlock explored this aspect of the driver aggression issue by correlating the number of road deaths with the number of violent deaths (murder and suicide) in numerous countries. From his research he concluded that road death and injury rates are the result, to a considerable extent, of the overall expression of aggressive behavior. Societies with the greatest amount of violence and aggression in their structure show this by externalizing some of this violence in the form of dangerous and aggressive driving.[85] Road rage and aggressive driving are then a reflection of larger societal problems.

Another driving concern these days, especially for urban commuters, is the dangerous combination of people talking on their cell phones while driving. There are around three hundred million cell phone subscribers in the U.S. It is estimated that 85% of cell phone owners use their phone while driving and that 60% of cell phone owner's usage occurs while driving.[86,87] Some cities have banned the use of cell phones while driving, but allow people to use hands-free devices. Because of safety concerns, several legislative efforts have been made to restrict cell phone use on the road. In most cases, the legislation regarding cell phones and driving focuses on limiting dialing or holding the phone while conversing. Research has shown that dialing the phone and answering the phone while driving does have a negative impact on driving.[88] However, the distracting effects of the phone conversation on driving are also considerable, and the duration of a typical phone conversation can be up to two orders of magnitude greater than the time required to dial or answer the phone.[89] Several studies have also found that working memory tasks and mental arithmetic tasks disrupt driving performance.[90] David Strayer, a University of Utah psychologist, has done a lot of cell phone research and has found that participants who engage in cell phone conversations are more likely to miss traffic signals and react to the signals more slowly than when they are not engaged in cell phone conversations.[91] The equivalent deficits in driving performance were obtained for both users of handheld and hands-free cell phones. His research showed that listening to radio broadcasts or books on tape, by contrast, did not impair driving performance. Other research has found impairments in the ability of participants to detect changes in real-world traffic scenes when they were conversing on a hands-free device; however, no such performance decrements were observed when participants listened to prerecorded conversations from other participants.[92] These findings demonstrate that listening to verbal material, by itself, is not sufficient to produce the dual-task interference associated with using a cell phone while driving. It seems that no matter how inane the conversations are there is a significant risk of talking while driving and such activity is responsible for a significant amount of automobile-related injury.

Carjacking is another motor vehicle related urban bodily harm concern. It is estimated that around 40,000 carjacking victimizations occur annually. Men were more often victimized than women; blacks more than whites; and Hispanics more than non-Hispanics. Households with annual incomes of $50,000 or more had lower rates than those making below $50,000, and carjacking victimization rates were highest in urban areas, followed by suburban and rural areas. Ninety-three percent of carjackings occurred in cities or suburbs. A weapon is used in 74% of carjacking victimizations; firearms were used in 45% of carjackings, knives in 11%, and other weapons in 18%. Victims often resist offenders. In the District of Columbia, between March 1 and mid-October 2020, carjackings and attempted carjackings jumped to 193 from 89 during the same period last year – a 117% increase. In Louisville, Kentucky, carjackings shot up during that same period from 68 to 194 – or 185%. Many of the victims are COVID-related food delivery drivers.

Automobiles and other forms of transportation are dangerous, and a significant source of bodily harm in the urban environment. A lot of people don't sense the danger and engage in activities (talking while driving, drinking while driving, and not wearing seatbelts) that get them into trouble. The other side of the equation is what fellow drivers are doing. One has to constantly be aware of what others are doing behind the wheel and also be cognizant of those who want to take someone's wheels.

Pedestrian and Cycling Injury

Walkin' in LA. Walkin' in LA, nobody walks in LA.
~ Missing Persons

And while driving is clearly dangerous, walking or riding bikes, unfortunately, can be dangerous too thanks in good part to automobiles. Each year in the United States around 900 bicyclists and 5,000 pedestrians are killed, and the majority of those killed are killed by cars. Walking or riding on roads with high speed limits and walking or riding at night increase the odds for a fatal injury. Head injury kills the majority of bicyclists and most fatally injured cyclists are over 20 years of age. The majority of all pedestrian crashes occur in urban areas where pedestrian activity and traffic volumes are greatest. The National Safety

Council estimates that 85.7% of all non-fatal pedestrian crashes in the United States occur in urban areas and 14.3% occur in rural areas. Seventy-two percent of all pedestrian fatalities occur in urban areas.[93] Most pedestrians are killed by cars or light trucks, but buses have a much higher pedestrian fatality per mile driven rate. In terms of crash location, 65% of crashes involving pedestrians occur at non-intersections – this is particularly true for pedestrians under age nine. For ages 45 to 65, pedestrian crashes are approximately equal for intersections and non-intersections. Pedestrians age 65 and older are more likely to be injured or killed at intersections (59%) compared to non-intersections (41%), since older pedestrians tend to cross at intersections more often than younger ones.[94] Pedestrian crashes are most prevalent during morning and afternoon peak periods, when the traffic levels are highest. Fatal pedestrian crashes typically peak later in the day, between 5 and 11pm, where darkness and alcohol use are factors. In 2003, 54% of the pedestrian fatalities occurred between 4pm and midnight. Nearly one-half of all pedestrian fatalities occurred on Friday, Saturday, or Sunday (16%, 18%, and 13%, respectively). Crashes where older pedestrians are hit are more evenly distributed throughout the days of the week than those for younger pedestrians. Older pedestrians are more likely to be struck during daylight hours, when they are most likely to be exposed to traffic. The highest number of pedestrian fatalities occurs between September through January principally due to fewer daylight hours and more inclement weather. Child pedestrian fatalities are greatest in May, June, and July, perhaps due to an increase in outside activity. Alcohol is a major contributing factor in pedestrian crashes. Of the 4,622 traffic crashes that resulted in a pedestrian fatality in 2003, 34% involved pedestrians with a blood-alcohol concentration (BAC) of 0.08 or greater. More than half of the pedestrian fatalities in the age groups of 21-24, 25-34, and 35 to 44 involved intoxicated pedestrians (55%, 57%, and 55%, respectively).[95]

Using data on average fatalities and population data, the NHTSA ranks large cities (with populations over a half million) based on their annual pedestrian fatality rates per year per 100,000 population. The following are the large cities with the best rates, along with their average annual pedestrian fatalities for the period:[96]

- Seattle, WA: Rate 1.01 (Fatalities: 6)
- Indianapolis, IN: Rate 1.09 (Fatalities: 9)
- Columbus, OH: Rate 1.41 (Fatalities: 10)
- Milwaukee, WI: Rate 1.45 (Fatalities: 9)
- Oklahoma City, OK: Rate 1.78 (Fatalities: 9)

The large cities with the highest pedestrian fatality rates were:

- Detroit, MI: Rate 5.05 (Fatalities: 48)
- Denver, CO: Rate 4.21 (Fatalities: 23)
- Phoenix, AZ: Rate 3.89 (Fatalities: 51)
- San Francisco, CA: Rate 3.82 (Fatalities: 30)
- Dallas, TX: Rate 3.51 (Fatalities: 42)

Work-Related Injury

The workplace is another significant source of bodily harm for urbanites. A lot of people spend a good proportion of their lives at work so it is only expected that at least some people would get hurt or killed in the workplace, but there are definitely some jobs that are more dangerous than others (liquor store clerk, cab driver, construction worker). There are a variety of workplaces in the city and thus many potential sources of bodily harm. Fatal highway incidents remained the most frequent type of fatal workplace event nationally, 2122 in 2019. Falls, slips, and trips fatalities were 880, and exposure to harmful substances or environments led to the deaths of 642 workers. In 2017, there were 458 workplace homicides. Of these, 77 were committed by coworkers or work associates, which accounted for the second largest assailant group behind robbery. This coworker assault is unfortunately becoming more common.

Though the home is typically thought of as a place to escape the dangers of the outside world, it ends up a significant source of bodily harm for urbanites. Every year around 20,000 people die and around 7 million sustain disabling injuries in the home in the U.S. Falls are the most common cause of injury in the home, but fires kill and injure a lot of people. Each year more than 4,000 Americans die and approximately 20,000 are injured in fires, many of which are preventable. Most fire-related deaths are caused by smoke inhalation. Smoking is the leading cause of fire-related deaths and cooking is the primary cause of residential fires.[97] Arson and malfunctioning heaters are other significant causes of fire-related death and injury. Approximately half of home fire deaths occur in homes without proper smoke alarms, and alcohol use contributes to an estimated 40% of residential fire deaths.[98] There have been several major fires that have impacted large U.S. cities over the years and one of the most significant fires was the 1871 Chicago fire, a.k.a, The Great Chicago Fire. The fire killed hundreds and destroyed several square miles, and was one of the largest U.S. disasters of the 19th century. The best-known story of the cause of the fire was that it was started by a cow kicking over a lantern in the barn owned by Patrick and Catherine O'Leary. Michael Ahern, the reporter who created the cow story for the newspaper, however, admitted in 1893 that he had made up the story because he thought it would make a colorful copy. The fire destroyed an area about four miles long encompassing more than 2,000 acres. The area included more than 73 miles of roads, 120 miles of sidewalk, 2,000 lampposts, 17,500 buildings, and $222 million in property – about a third of the city's valuation. Out of 300,000 inhabitants, 100,000 were left homeless.[99] While much has been done to prevent catastrophes of this proportion – alarms, building materials – these events still occur.

In urban settings, fires that occur in densely populated buildings (high rises) can be especially problematic. High rise fires pose significant problems for both fire suppression and occupant safety. When buildings are constructed beyond the reach of a fire department's highest ladder, two important firefighting strategies are taken away from firefighters. First, life-saving victim removals using ladders are eliminated. Searches and rescues can be accomplished only from inside stairways. The second firefighting strategy that is taken away is the ability to extinguish a fire with an outside master stream – firefighters are forced to extinguish the fire using handheld hose streams advanced through heat and smoke from an inside stairway. Other high rise fire issues are lack of functioning routes of escape, poor emergency preparedness planning, and alarm and sprinkling system problems.[100] The 1980 MGM Grand fire in Las Vegas showed what happens when a fire occurs in a crowded building. Mass panic ensues and whatever safeguards and plans are in place are soon forgotten. Eighty-five people died, mostly because of smoke inhalation. How prepared is your building or home to handle a fire?

Building Integrity
The collapse of the Champlain Towers South condo building in Florida on June 24, 2021 brought the issue of structural integrity of high rise buildings to the forefront. Most of us believe when we are in high rises that they are structurally sound; they passed some test; someone checked them. Obviously, not.

The 12-story beachfront condominium collapsed killing 98 people. Sure, the building did have some inspections over the years with some findings, but no one compelled the owners to evacuate and repair. The metal and concrete structural elements basically had disintegrated. Living in a tent somehow now seems so much safer.

Terrorism

Finally, and perhaps most significantly, terrorism has become another potential source of bodily harm in urban America. The terrorist attacks of 9/11/01 forever changed the landscape of big city life in the U.S. Subsequent similar attacks on trains in London and Madrid reinforced the idea that the potential of being a victim of a terrorist attack is a part of the city violence equation. While thousands of people die each year in the U.S. as a result of accidents and homicides, the 9/11 events continue to trump all in the minds of many. 2,973 people were killed, including 246 on the four planes, 2,602 in New York City in the towers and on the ground, and 125 at the Pentagon as a result of the attacks. Among the fatalities were 343 New York City Fire Department firefighters, 23 New York City Police Department officers, and 37 Port Authority police officers.[101] On June 12, 2016, 29-year-old Omar Mateen killed 49 people and wounded 58 others in a mass shooting at a dance club in Orlando. The attack was the deadliest single gunman mass shooting in United States history until the 2017 Las Vegas shooting where 61 concertgoers were killed. Being part of a crowd, makes you part of the crowd when those with deadly intent want to randomly kill lots of people.

Chapter 5

Infectious Diseases

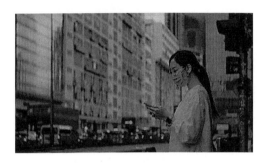

Infectious Diseases

An illness is like a journey into a far country; it sifts all one's experience and removes it to a point so remote that it appears like a vision.

~ Sholem Asch

Infectious or communicable diseases are human illnesses caused by viruses, bacteria, parasites, fungi and other microbes. They may be spread by direct contact with an infected person or animal, by ingesting contaminated food or water, by insects like mosquitoes or ticks, or by contact with contaminated surroundings like animal droppings or even contaminated air. Many people get infections, but not everyone who gets an infection becomes ill. Disease occurs only when the causative agent comes into contact with a susceptible host in a suitable environment. The most worrisome infectious agents, especially for city dwellers, are those that are both very contagious and virulent; lethal diseases that can spread quickly through a crowded community. COVID.

Near the time of the publication of this book, there were

close to 200 million cases of COVID and near four million deaths worldwide. Twenty-five million cases and nearly 500,000 deaths in the United States. Where did it come from? Most likely China. Was it natural or man-made? Unclear, likely man-made. COVID, COVID-19 in this instance, is a Coronavirus. It's not all that unusual. They, like rhinoviruses, can cause the common cold. They can also jump from animals to humans like it did with SARS 15 years ago. The SARS epidemic of 2004 demonstrated how quickly things could go awry when an infectious disease threat shows up. The outbreak in Toronto demonstrated how quickly an infectious disease can derail business activities; overwhelm hospitals and the public health system; and lead to discriminatory practices and widespread panic. This was a precursor to COVID; a taste of what was possible, a warning shot. We were given a chance to prepare and did little, and did not take the threat seriously enough when it arrived. We at one point had stockpiled millions and millions of masks years before COVID. And then we sold them, some to China. This COVID is not the last COVID. This deadly infectious disease will certainly not be the last. While COVID has made it to all corners of the globe, it started in highly populated areas and that's where the majority of cases have occurred.

At this point, we all know that COVID causes a respiratory infection that taxes the lungs – severe infections lead to respiratory failure and death. COVID also does the following damage and related problems both during acute infection and beyond:

Fatigue
Shortness of breath
Cough
Joint pain
Chest pain
Difficulty with thinking and concentration

Depression

Muscle pain

Headache

Intermittent fever

Fast-beating or pounding heart

Hair loss

Insomnia

The great flu pandemic of 1918 killed millions worldwide. Several infectious diseases have plagued urban environs in the past (tuberculosis, bubonic plague), and there are concerns that revamped old "bugs" will cause problems again. Human history and infectious diseases are deeply intertwined. Tuberculosis was the leading cause of death followed by pneumonia and diarrhea in the United States in 1900. Along with diphtheria these conditions accounted for more than 30% of all deaths in the country.[102] Since then major reductions in morbidity and mortality from communicable diseases have resulted from improvements in sanitation, housing, and nutrition as well as introduction and use of vaccines and specific therapies. Improvements in sanitation have dramatically reduced the burden of water- and foodborne diseases. Improvements in housing played an important role in reducing transmission of tuberculosis, and improvements in nutrition have made persons with infectious diseases less likely to die from their infections.

The introduction and use of vaccines have resulted in global eradication of smallpox, significant progress toward eradication of polio, and a marked reduction in illness and death due to diseases such as diphtheria, whooping cough (pertussis), and measles. Specific therapies such as antibiotics and antiparasitic drugs have had a significant impact on deaths due to infectious diseases as well as having some impact on the occurrence of the diseases by shortening the period in which an infected person is infectious to others. While there has been some success in the war against the bugs since 1900 it appears that the bugs aren't going away anytime soon. Infectious diseases, once thought to be almost eliminated as a public health problem, remain the leading cause of death worldwide. Approximately half of all world deaths caused by infectious diseases each year can be attributed to just three infectious diseases: tuberculosis, malaria, and AIDS.[103] Together, these diseases cause over 300 million illnesses and more than 5 million deaths each year worldwide. Infectious diseases kill well over 100,000 Americans annually and they account for around 25% of all physician visits each year. Around 35,000 people in the United States die from the flu alone each year. And, over the past 20 years, some new bugs – West Nile, SARS, Mad Cow, and Bird Flu – have surfaced and have caused their share of problems and threaten to cause even more illness and death.

One's susceptibility to infectious diseases depends on many factors such as where one lives, who they live with, age, general health, and activities. Infectious diseases tend to be regionalized, but every so often they "jump the fence." In some parts of the world, for example, certain diseases such as malaria and cholera are constantly present in an area (they are endemic); in other parts of the world these diseases pose little or no threat at all. Urban environs, unfortunately, are particularly good breeding and spreading grounds for infectious diseases due to a variety of factors such as high population density and urban lifestyles that are often associated with a higher incidence of infectious disease. And it also appears that terrorists have their sights set on cities; city dwellers are now also at risk of having infectious diseases like smallpox and anthrax used as weapons against them. Some have argued that COVID was a targeted attack by China; we don't have evidence of that. Most infectious diseases, however, typically don't go out of their way to "get" people except for the very young and the very old. A lot of people who get sick from infectious diseases have some responsibility for their own illness. People who smoke; abuse drugs and alcohol; have unprotected sex; don't exercise; don't seek healthcare; and don't get immunized put themselves at risk of acquiring infections. Those who ran around without a mask during COVID put themselves and others at risk.

A Brief History of Infectious Diseases

Over the past few hundred years we have come to understand that illness and death can be caused by living organisms that we cannot see. Prior to a few hundred years ago most people attributed such illnesses to witchcraft or other cosmic forces. The bubonic plague or the "Black Death" which began in China's Gobi Desert in the 1300s and killed 35 million in Western Europe and around the same in Asia is perhaps the most well-known infectious disease calamity. The disease is believed to have been caused by the *Yersinia pestis* bacterium which passed from infected rats to humans via fleas. While people at that time weren't sure what was causing the illness some people were at least aware that you could "catch it" from others. Leeuwenhoek's discovery of bacteria via the microscope in the 1600s was the critical first step in the understanding of the role of microscopic organisms in causing illness and death. Scientists later realized that these bacteria or "germs" could be spread person to person and via contaminated water supplies. Edward Jenner discovered that sometimes exposure to one disease could protect one from another disease. In the late eighteen hundreds Koch and Pasteur helped further advance the germ theory of disease. Scientists concluded that microorganisms were responsible for a variety of illnesses near the end of the nineteenth century. From the early to the mid-1900s more advances were made in bacteriology and virology including the development of the polio vaccine and antibiotics. Death rates from infectious and parasitic diseases declined during the late 19th century and throughout most of the 20th century thanks to better public health and sanitation as well as medical advances made possible by economic development.[104] Infectious disease mortality declined (except during the flu pandemic of 1918) during the first seven decades of the 20th century from 797 deaths per 100,000 in 1900 to 36 deaths per 100,000 in 1970. From 1938 to 1952, the decline was particularly rapid, with mortality decreasing 8.2% per year.[105] When smallpox was eradicated from the globe in the late 1970s many health experts believed that infectious and parasitic diseases could at long last be conquered. It looked as though the "bugs" were finally losing the battle, but then HIV showed up in the early eighties. Infectious disease mortality then increased in the 1980s and early 1990s. Although most of the 20th century was marked by declining infectious disease mortality, recent COVID increases and episodes of higher mortality demonstrate that infectious diseases are still a problem.

Specifically, more than 100 "new" or previously unrecognized disease-causing microbes have been identified since 1973. The Institute of Medicine (IOM) of the National Academy of Sciences' 1992 report, *Emerging Infections: Microbial Threats to Health in the United States*, concluded that emerging infectious diseases are a major threat to U.S. health, and it challenged the U.S. government to take action.[106] As defined in the 1992 Institute of Medicine report, emerging infectious diseases include diseases whose incidence in humans has increased within the past two decades or threaten to increase in the near future. Modern demographic and environmental conditions that favor the spread of these emerging infectious diseases include:

- Global travel;
- Globalization of the food supply and centralized processing of food; population growth and increased urbanization and crowding;
- Population movements due to civil wars, famines, and other man-made or natural disasters;

- Irrigation, deforestation, and reforestation projects that alter the habitats of disease-carrying insects and animals;
- Human behaviors, such as intravenous drug use and risky sexual behavior;
- Increased use of antimicrobial agents and pesticides, hastening the development of resistance;
- Increased human contact with tropical rainforests and other wilderness habitats that are reservoirs for insects and animals that harbor unknown infectious agents.

New disease agents and revamped old ones have already caused their share of problems and more of these "super bugs" are expected to arrive in the years to come. It seems that infectious diseases will continue to plague humans, especially those living in urban environments.

Infectious Diseases 101

Infectious diseases spread via three mechanisms: direct transmission, indirect transmission, and through airborne transmission. Direct transmission refers to direct contact such as touching, biting, kissing, sexual intercourse, or the direct projection of droplet spray into the eye, nose, or mouth during sneezing, coughing, spitting, singing, or talking. The easiest way to catch most infectious diseases is by coming into direct contact with someone who has one. Pets can also transmit infections via bites, scratches and through handling their waste. And a pregnant woman can pass infectious diseases (HIV, toxoplasmosis) on to an unborn baby via the placenta or they can be passed during labor and delivery.

Indirect transmission can occur through a vehicle (food, water) or through insects like mosquitoes, ticks and fleas. Some infectious organisms rely on insects to move from host to host. These insect carriers are known as vectors. Mosquitoes can carry the malaria parasite or West Nile virus and deer ticks carry the bacterium that causes Lyme disease. The vector-borne spread of a disease happens when an insect that carries an organism on its body or in its intestinal tract lands on a person or bites them. Infectious disease vehicles include water, food, biological products, or contaminated articles (such as syringes). Water and foodborne diseases, of course, have the potential for causing outbreaks involving thousands of persons. Common-vehicle transmissions like tainted salad from a large manufacturer allow organisms to be spread to many people through a single source. Before the causative agent was identified, many cases of HIV resulted from blood transfusion – blood was the vehicle of transmission. Disease-causing organisms can also be passed through inanimate objects like tables and doorknobs. When a person touches the same doorknob grasped by someone ill with the flu or a cold or COVID, for example, they can pick up the germs left behind. If that person then touches their eyes, mouth or nose before washing their hands, they may become infected.

Infectious diseases can also be spread via the air. Airborne spread requires that infectious particles (droplets) are small enough to be suspended in the air long enough to be inhaled by the recipient. Crowded, indoor environments are ideal environments for such droplet transmission thus explaining the increase in respiratory infections in the winter months and during the COVID pandemic. Diseases like tuberculosis can be spread in this fashion. Airborne transmission can also be used to disseminate agents of biological warfare or bioterrorism.

For most communicable diseases there is an interval between infection and occurrence of symptoms (the incubation period) in which the infectious agent is multiplying or developing. Some persons who are infected may never develop manifestations of the disease even though they may be capable of transmitting it. Some persons may carry (and transmit) the agent over prolonged periods (carriers) whether or not they develop symptoms. Treatment during the incubation period may cure the infection, thereby preventing both disease and transmission. This preventive treatment (chemoprophylaxis) is often used in persons who have been exposed to sexually transmitted diseases such as syphilis and gonorrhea. It also is effective in persons who have been infected with tuberculosis.[107]

The sociocultural environment is another important factor in the spread of communicable diseases. HIV, for example, rapidly spread through some communities because of sexual practices and intravenous (IV) drug use and has been relatively absent from others. Social influences, in turn, have reduced HIV infection rates in communities through the promotion of condom use; the use of condoms during anal intercourse, for example, was not a common practice prior to the AIDS era. Public health practices in particular can influence the sociocultural environment and the spread of communicable diseases. Public health practices include safe water and food laws, provision of free immunization and chemoprophylaxis through public health departments, enactment and enforcement of school immunization requirements, isolation of individuals with communicable diseases to prevent transmission, and quarantine of individuals exposed to communicable diseases to prevent disease transmission during the incubation period if they have been infected. The role of the public health departments took prominence during the COVID pandemic – many were calling the shots around lockdowns and other activities. Educating people to properly cook food, wash hands, and sterilize surgical instruments are other public health interventions. The proper treatment of sewage and handling of trash are also important measures. The use of respiratory protective devices (PPE) in hospital settings (and others) can be used to prevent passage of microorganisms into the respiratory tract. And reduction of crowding and appropriate ventilation also reduces the likelihood of droplet or airborne transmission of infectious diseases.

Antibiotics have been one of the main and most important

weapons used to fight infections over the past 60 years. While great strides have been made using antibiotics (including antivirals and antifungals) to treat infectious diseases, the causative organisms often become resistant to the antibiotics. Antibiotics have, in fact, been overused over the years and such overuse has led to the creation of superbugs. Staphylococcus aureus is one such superbug and is a major problem in the hospital environment. It became resistant to penicillin first and then it became resistant to methicillin and then it became resistant to vancomycin (a very powerful antibiotic).[108] Because strains of the bacterium are now resistant to almost everything there is almost nothing that can be done to stop it once a person is infected. The same progression toward resistance has occurred with tuberculosis and there are many throughout the world who are infected with and dying from multidrug-resistant tuberculosis.

Vaccines have also been used and continue to be used to battle infectious diseases and have done much to limit and even eradicate some diseases. Vaccines work by stimulating the immune system to develop antibodies and thus engage the body in the fight against the intruder. The immune system recognizes vaccine agents as foreign, destroys them, and remembers them. When the virulent version of an agent comes along, the immune system is thus prepared to respond, by neutralizing the target agent before it can enter cells, and by recognizing and destroying infected cells before that agent can multiply to vast numbers. Edward Jenner, an English physician, is often credited with the discovery of vaccines because of his observation in 1796 that those who caught cowpox (a milder form of smallpox) developed immunity against smallpox. Jenner then intentionally infected a boy with cowpox and later exposed him to smallpox and he did not develop the disease. Today's vaccines are now made up of inactivated or attenuated strains of viruses or bacteria; their components; or are completely synthetic. The COVID vaccine uses messenger RNA to infect cells and produce part of the shell of the virus. The body sees that foreign protein and creates antibodies against it. Vaccines have contributed to the eradication of smallpox, one of the most contagious and deadly diseases known to man. Other diseases such as rubella, polio, measles, mumps, chickenpox, and typhoid are nowhere near as common as they were just a hundred years ago.[109] Vaccines are now also being used to fight some types of cancer and a vaccine for HIV continues to be worked on. COVID vaccines have been developed. But vaccines are not entirely free of controversy. Some believe that vaccines are responsible for diseases like autism yet no firm connection has been made. Some communities refuse to vaccinate their children because of such beliefs. And sometimes, vaccines simply don't work.

Cities and Infectious Diseases

Since the city is, by definition, the place where human density is greatest, it is not surprising that cities have spawned epidemics. One only has to imagine someone "coughing their lungs out" on a crowded subway train and it's not difficult to conceptualize how one person's cough could become everyone's epidemic. Human plagues such as the Black Death, cholera, tuberculosis (TB), and HIV are essentially the by-products of urban living. Crowded conditions in urban areas continue to provide an ideal environment for the culture and spread of old diseases like TB as well as for many newly emerging diseases. Certain infections such as TB and meningitis are especially adept at spreading rather easily through high-population density settings (e.g., day care centers or prisons).[110] In order for an epidemic to occur there has to be a certain threshold density of susceptible individuals. In addition to the effects of increased human contact on disease transmission, demographics may also influence other environmental factors relevant to disease emergence. For example, crowded urban settings or unanticipated mass migrations can overburden sanitation systems and create conditions that allow the introduction and spread of foodborne and waterborne organisms. The reappearance of plague, cholera, and dengue in many parts of the world is due in part to the rapid growth of impoverished peri-urban areas around "mega-cities" that lack appropriate sanitation. These problems are expected to only worsen as the world population doubles in the next 30 years.[111]

City dwellers do in fact face increased infectious disease risk because of factors such as close contact with others; inadequate public health surveillance; higher prevalence of certain behaviorally-related diseases such as HIV; more global visitors, residents, and trade; more contact with rodents and other disease vectors; higher percentage consumption of food from outside of the home; and the lack of adequate healthcare for many residents. While foreign terrorist activities involving biological agents are another potential source of infectious disease concern no confirmed such activity has yet occurred. The post 9/11 anthrax attacks in 2001 that killed five people remain a mystery, but so far it seems that they were not caused by terrorists per se and also demonstrated how difficult it is to cause mass casualties using most biological weapons.[112]

There are many ways for an infectious disease to enter into, gain hold, and spread throughout a city. One such way is through the introduction of a previously unknown organism that residents have no immunity against. History is replete with examples of such imported infections. Trade between Asia and Europe in the thirteenth and fourteenth centuries brought the rat and one of its infections, the bubonic plague, to Europe. Beginning in the 16th and 17th centuries, ships bringing slaves from West Africa to the New World also brought yellow fever and its mosquito vector, Aedes aegypti, to the new territories. Similarly, smallpox escaped its Old World origins to wreak new havoc in the New World. In the 19th century, cholera had similar opportunities to spread from its probable origin in the Ganges plain to the Middle East and, from there, to Europe and much of the remaining world. Similar occurrences are being repeated today, but opportunities in recent years have become far richer and more numerous, reflecting the increasing volume, scope, and speed of traffic in an increasingly mobile world. Rats have carried hantaviruses virtually worldwide. *Aedes albopictus* (the Asian tiger mosquito) was introduced into the United States, Brazil, and parts of Africa in shipments of used tires from Asia. Since its introduction in 1982, this mosquito has established itself in at least 18 states of the United States and has acquired local viruses including Eastern equine encephalomyelitis, a cause of serious disease. Another mosquito-borne disease, malaria, is one of the most frequently imported diseases in non-endemic-disease areas, and now seems to spreading to other parts of the world.[113] And we have the tale of COVID to add to the mix. It's pretty clear the infection started in Wuhan, China and worked its way across the globe. A Chinese national who landed in Seattle may have got things cooking in the United States and it just took off. Exotic infectious diseases continue to be brought into cities worldwide by those migrating from rural to urban environs; in the U.S. infectious diseases are brought into the city by those from other countries who are visiting or by natives returning from their travels. The bottom line is that we live in a very global world and urbanites are typically a very globe-trotting set. One can easily acquire an illness in another part of the world and come home with it before showing any signs of illness.

While recent immigrants are certainly not entirely responsible for infectious disease outbreaks in the U.S., they can be an important source of infectious disease. Individuals born outside the United States accounted for 46% of the 16,377 U.S. cases of tuberculosis (TB) reported in 2000.[114] Tuberculosis screening is required for immigrants who apply for citizenship, but no such screening is done for those who do not apply for citizenship – no formal screening is done at airports or other ports of entry. A total of 9,029 new cases of TB were reported in the United States in 2018, which was a 0.7% decrease from 2017. The decrease in incidence from 2017 to 2018 was 1.3%. The rate in non-US-born citizens was >14-fold greater than that in US-born citizens and non-US-born persons accounted for approximately two-thirds of cases.

International commerce is another potential source of infectious disease as foods and other products from other countries make it to the marketplace and may harbor organisms capable of causing illness. An outbreak of cholera in South America, for example, was determined to be from contaminated bilge water from an Asian freighter.[115] New bacterial strains, such as the recently identified Vibrio cholerae O139, or an epidemic strain of *Neisseria meningitidis* (the cause of meningitis), have disseminated rapidly along routes of trade and travel, as have antibiotic-resistant bacteria.[116] Food is another important source of infectious disease and a lot of the food consumed in the U.S. comes from other countries. Such food is either not screened or poorly screened for pathogens.

Public health departments are chiefly responsible for limiting the spread of communicable diseases in U.S. cities. And while all big cities have public health departments, many are simply unprepared and do not have the funding to adequately respond to large infectious disease outbreaks as we saw with COVID. The outbreak of the waterborne Cryptosporidium infection in Milwaukee, Wisconsin, in the spring of 1993, with over 400,000 estimated cases, was in part due to a nonfunctioning water filtration plant – a public health function.[117] Similar deficiencies in water purification have been found in other cities in the United States, and maintaining a water supply that is free of infectious organisms is a critical public health responsibility especially in a large city where many are totally dependent on municipal water. Over three trillion dollars are spent on healthcare in the United States each year yet it is estimated that less than 1% of the money goes to support public health activities.[118] And local public health departments are increasingly being called upon to provide basic medical services further diminishing their capacity to concentrate on and prevent infectious disease outbreaks. Another urban issue is, of course, the relatively high level of uninsured residents. People without insurance often delay seeking treatment when ill and thus can be another significant source of infectious disease dissemination.

Behavior, especially sexual and drug-related, is also responsible for the spread of infectious diseases, and rates of IV drug use and unsafe sexual practices (prostitutes, multiple partners) are often much higher in urban environs. Twenty-five percent of people with HIV/AIDS are IV drug users. Another significant source of HIV infection for women is sex with partners who are IDUs. An estimated 61% of AIDS cases in women can be attributed to injecting drug use or to sex with partners who are IDUs.

Diseases of Concern

While there are many infectious diseases that are more common in urban environments, all urbanites are at risk of illness as a result of exposure to a variety of infectious diseases. People naturally fear the bugs they hear most about (COVID, bird flu, flesh-eating bacteria, Ebola, mad cow) but, aside from HIV in certain cities, it is the non-exotic infections (flu, bacterial pneumonia) that are the big killers.

Disease Traffickers

It is well established that asthma and allergies can be caused by and exacerbated by exposure to dust mites, cockroaches, pets, and rodents, but such animals can also spread disease, and there are plenty of bugs and animals in urban environs.

There are more than 200 diseases of animals transmissible to people (zoonoses) causing a wide variety of human illness.[119] Twenty-one human infectious disease outbreaks associated with animals in public settings occurred between 1990 and 2000 in the U.S. Since 2001, 35 additional outbreaks have occurred in the United States.[120] Rodents (rats and mice) are well known for their ability to spread infectious disease. Rats are thought to have been responsible for the bubonic plague which killed over 20 million people. Rodent-related diseases affecting humans include plague, typhus, leptospirosis, rickettsialpox, and rat-bite fever.[121] A CDC survey of two major American cities documented that nearly 50% of the premises were inhabited by rats and mice, especially deer mice.[122] Hantavirus is another infectious disease spread by rodents. Hantavirus causes a severe respiratory illness. It is spread to people when they breathe in dust that contains the rodents' infected saliva, urine or feces. As of September 2004, a total of 379 laboratory-confirmed cases of hantavirus disease had been reported in the United States, primarily in the Southwest. Thirty-six percent of all reported cases have resulted in death.[123]

Cockroaches are another ubiquitous pest in the urban world. Although little evidence exists to link cockroaches to specific disease outbreaks, they have been demonstrated to harbor several significant bugs, Salmonella and the polio virus. There is some thought that cockroaches might also be able to spread diseases like SARS or COVID. Fleas can also spread disease including typhus and bubonic plague. In addition, fleas serve as intermediate hosts for some species of dog and rodent tapeworms that occasionally infest people. Flies are another significant source of infectious diseases. A housefly can easily carry more than 1 million bacteria on its body. Some of the disease-causing agents transmitted by houseflies to humans are Shigella (a cause of dysentery and diarrhea), Salmonella (diarrhea and typhoid fever), Escherichia coli (traveler's diarrhea), and Vibrio cholera (cholera). Mosquitoes are another significant source of infectious disease especially in Third World countries where they are responsible for millions of malaria deaths each year. Mosquito-borne diseases, such as malaria and yellow fever, have plagued civilization for thousands of years. Mosquitoes continue to spread a variety of diseases across the world and carry new threats like the bacterium that causes Lyme disease and the West Nile Virus.[124]

While dogs and cats often make great companions they can also make people sick. The population of companion animals continues to increase with approximately one person in five owning at least one animal.[125] Cats can transmit Cat Scratch Disease – a bacterial disease that invades lymph nodes, and toxoplasmosis – a parasitic disease that can kill people who are immunocompromised and harm a developing fetus.[126] Animals, especially dogs and other wild animals like squirrels, can infect humans with rabies though such cases are now very rare.

The Flu and Pneumonia

Over fifty thousand people die each year as a result of influenza (flu) and pneumonia. Pneumonia and influenza together are ranked as the seventh leading cause of death in the United States. Pneumonia consistently accounts for the overwhelming majority of deaths between the two. The vast majority (75%) of flu and pneumonia deaths occurred in the elderly – especially those over the age of 75. Pneumonia is an inflammation of the lung caused by infection with bacteria, viruses, and other organisms. Pneumonia is often a complication of a preexisting condition or infection, and it occurs when a patient's defense system is weakened, most often by a simple viral upper respiratory tract infection or a case of influenza. The bacterium *Streptococcus pneumoniae* (also known as pneumococcal pneumonia) is the most common cause of pneumonia acquired outside of hospitals. The bacteria can multiply and cause serious damage to healthy individual lungs, bloodstream (bacteremia), brain (meningitis) and other parts of the body, especially when the body's defenses are weakened. Pneumococcal pneumonia accounts for 25 to 35 percent of all community-acquired pneumonia, and an estimated 40,000 deaths yearly. People considered at high risk for pneumonia include the elderly, the very young, and those with underlying health problems, such as chronic obstructive pulmonary disease (COPD), diabetes mellitus, congestive heart failure and sickle cell anemia. Patients with diseases that impair the immune system, such as AIDS, or those undergoing cancer therapy or organ transplantation, or patients with other chronic illnesses are particularly vulnerable.[127] Hospitals are another important source of pneumonia in the U.S. There is an immunization to prevent bacterial pneumonia (the pneumococcal vaccine, not the flu shot). The flu is a contagious respiratory illness caused by influenza viruses and the flu season typically runs from November to April. The flu can cause mild to severe illness, and at times can lead to death. Every year in the United States 5% to 20% of the population gets the flu; more than 200,000 people are hospitalized from flu complications, and about 36,000 people die from flu. Many people who have a cold think they have the flu. Flu symptoms include:

- High fever
- Headache
- Fatigue
- Dry cough
- Sore throat and stuffy nose
- Muscle aches
- Nausea, vomiting, and diarrhea

Flu viruses spread mainly from person to person through coughing or sneezing of people with influenza. Sometimes people may become infected by touching something with flu viruses on it and then touching their mouth or nose. Most healthy adults may be able to infect others beginning one day before symptoms develop and up to five days after becoming sick.[128] There are three types of influenza viruses: A, B, and C. Subtypes of influenza A that are currently circulating among people worldwide include H1N1, H1N2, and H3N2 viruses. Wild birds are the natural host for all known subtypes of influenza A viruses. Wild birds do not become sick when they are infected with influenza A viruses, but domestic poultry, such as turkeys and chickens, can become very sick and die from influenza A. Influenza viruses are dynamic and are continuously evolving. Influenza viruses can change in two different ways: antigenic drift and antigenic shift. Antigenic drift refers to small, gradual changes that occur through mutations in the genes that contain the genetic material to produce the main surface proteins of the influenza virus. Antigenic shift refers to an abrupt, major change that produces a novel influenza A virus subtype in humans that was not currently circulating. Antigenic shift can occur either through direct animal (poultry)-to-human transmission or through mixing of human influenza A and animal influenza A virus genes to create a new human influenza. It is these types of changes that are most worrisome as a strain of the virus could be created that humans have no immunity against. There is, fortunately, a flu vaccine and around 60% of the U.S. population gets the vaccine each year. Vaccines typically contain three attenuated influenza viruses. Each of the three vaccine strains in both vaccines – one A (H3N2) virus, one A (H1N1) virus, and one B virus – are used in the batch of flu vaccine that is produced each year.[129]

Foodborne Illness

People, in general, and city dwellers in particular, consume a lot of food that is not prepared in the home. It is estimated that people now eat nearly 60% of their meals outside of the home.[130]

In places like Manhattan, ordering in Chinese is a fairly regular activity and many source their meals from local delis and markets. While cities have restaurant inspection programs and the CDC monitors outbreaks, such programs don't guarantee food safety. Foodborne disease is caused by consuming contaminated foods or beverages. Many different disease-causing microbes, or pathogens, can contaminate foods, so there are many different foodborne infections. In addition, poisonous chemicals, or other harmful substances can cause foodborne diseases if they are present in food. These different diseases have many different symptoms, so there is no one "syndrome" that is foodborne illness; the symptoms produced depend greatly on the type of microbe. Nausea, vomiting, abdominal cramps and diarrhea are signs of foodborne illness. It is difficult to determine which organism is involved unless laboratory tests are done to identify the microbe, or unless the illness is part of a recognized outbreak. Foodborne diseases cause approximately 76 million illnesses, 325,000 hospitalizations, and 5,000 deaths in the United States each year. Foodborne illness can be especially deadly for the young, elderly, and the immunocompromised. Known pathogens account for an estimated 14 million illnesses, 60,000 hospitalizations, and 1,800 deaths. Three pathogens, Salmonella, Listeria, and Toxoplasma, are "responsible for 1,500 deaths each year, more than 75% of those caused by known pathogens, while unknown agents account for the remaining 62 million illnesses, 265,000 hospitalizations, and 3,200 deaths." According to the CDC, the following factors contribute to foodborne illness:[131]

- Inadequate Cooling and Cold Holding Temperatures
- Preparing Food Ahead of Planned Service
- Inadequate Holding Temperatures
- Poor Personal Hygiene/Infected Persons
- Inadequate Reheating

- Inadequate Cleaning of Equipment
- Use of Leftovers
- Cross-Contamination
- Contaminated Raw Ingredients

The most commonly recognized foodborne infections are those caused by the bacteria Campylobacter, Salmonella, and E. coli O157:H7, and by a group of viruses known as Norwalk viruses.[132] Campylobacter is the most commonly identified bacterial cause of diarrheal illness in the world. Campylobacter lives in the intestines of healthy birds, and most raw poultry meat has Campylobacter on it. Eating undercooked chicken, or other food that has been contaminated with juices dripping from raw chicken is the most frequent source of this infection.[133] Salmonella infection is another common foodborne illness and it can be especially dangerous for those with poor underlying health or weakened immune systems as it can invade the bloodstream and cause life-threatening infections. Salmonella lives in the intestinal tracts of humans and other animals, including birds. Salmonella are usually transmitted to humans by eating foods contaminated with animal feces. Salmonella-contaminated foods usually look and smell normal. The foods are often of animal origin, such as beef, poultry, milk, or eggs, but all foods, including vegetables, may become contaminated. While many raw foods of animal origin are frequently contaminated, thorough cooking kills Salmonella. Food may also become contaminated by the unwashed hands of an infected food handler. Salmonella may also be found in the feces of some pets, especially those with diarrhea, and people can become infected if they do not wash their hands after contact with these feces. Reptiles are particularly likely to harbor Salmonella.[134] E. coli O157:H7 is a bacterial pathogen that has a reservoir in cattle and other similar animals. Human illness typically follows consumption of food or water that has been contaminated with microscopic amounts of cow feces. E. coli causes a severe and bloody diarrhea and painful abdominal cramps, without much fever. Though most illness has been associated with eating undercooked, contaminated ground beef, people have also become ill from eating contaminated bean sprouts or fresh leafy vegetables such as lettuce and spinach. Person-to-person contact in families and child care centers is also a known mode of transmission.[135]

Hepatitis A (HAV) is another significant cause of foodborne illness though it can also be contracted through sexual contact or via contaminated water. Around 250,000 HAV infections occur each year. Hepatitis A begins with symptoms such as fever, anorexia, nausea, vomiting, diarrhea, myalgia, and malaise. Jaundice, dark-colored urine, or light-colored stools might be present at onset or might follow constitutional symptoms within a few days. For most persons, hepatitis A lasts for several weeks. Food handlers are often responsible for many hepatitis A outbreaks each year.[136] Toxoplasmosis is a ubiquitous parasite that causes foodborne illness and serious disease for those who are pregnant or immunocompromised. It is estimated that around 60 million people are infected with toxoplasmosis.[137] And finally, Listeria is another fairly common foodborne illness. Listeria is found in soil and water and vegetables can become contaminated from the soil or from manure used as fertilizer. Animals can carry the bacterium without appearing ill and can contaminate foods of animal origin such as meats and dairy products. The bacterium has been found in a variety of raw foods, such as uncooked meats and vegetables, as well as in processed foods that become contaminated after processing, such as soft cheeses and cold cuts at the deli counter. Unpasteurized (raw) milk or foods made from unpasteurized milk may contain the bacterium. Listeria is killed by pasteurization and cooking; however, in certain ready-to-eat foods such as hot dogs and deli meats, contamination may occur after cooking but before packaging.[138]

Waterborne Illness

Most waterborne illness in the U.S. occurs as a result of recreational exposures, but there are occasional outbreaks due to contaminated drinking water. Drinking water pathogens include bacteria, viruses and parasitic protozoa (another type of infectious organism). Bacteria and viruses contaminate both surface and groundwater, whereas parasitic protozoa appear predominantly in surface water. All municipal water is treated in the U.S. to kill or inactivate microorganisms so that they cannot reproduce and infect human hosts. Bacteria and viruses are well-controlled by normal chlorination, in contrast to parasitic protozoa, which demand more sophisticated control measures. From 1991 to 2000, there were 155 outbreaks and 431,846 cases of illness in public and individual U.S. water systems. The largest outbreak of this period occurred in 1993 with the Cryptosporidium in Milwaukee when over 400,000 people got sick.[139]

Sexually Transmitted Infections

There are many infectious diseases that are spread through sexual contact (sexually transmitted infections of STI) including herpes, hepatitis, gonorrhea, chlamydia, syphilis, human papilloma virus and most significantly, HIV. As noted before, STI and HIV rates are often much higher in the urban world. It is estimated that nearly a million Americans (mostly urbanites) are living with human immunodeficiency virus (HIV) infection. In 2004, the estimated number of deaths of persons with AIDS was 15,798, including 15,737 adults and adolescents, and 61 children under age 13. The cumulative estimated number of deaths of persons with AIDS through 2004 was 529,113, including 523,598 adults and adolescents, and 5,515 children under age 13. HIV infection rates remain high, especially among minority populations and gay males. Of newly diagnosed HIV infections in the United States the CDC estimated that approximately 67%

were among men who were infected through sexual contact with other men, 50% were among blacks, 32% were among whites, and 16% were among Hispanics.[140] A study that involved random HIV testing of gay males in five U.S. cities showed that 25% were HIV positive and nearly 50% were not aware that they were infected. In 2018, there were 15,820 deaths among adults and adolescents with diagnosed HIV in the U.S. and dependent areas. These deaths may be due to any cause. Heterosexuals continue to be affected by HIV. In 2018, heterosexuals accounted for 24% of the 37,968 new HIV diagnoses.[141]

HIV is spread by sexual contact with an infected person, by sharing needles and/or syringes (primarily for drug injection) with someone who is infected. Babies born to HIV-infected women may become infected before or during birth or through breast-feeding after birth. In the healthcare setting, workers have been infected with HIV (and other bloodborne pathogens) after being stuck with needles containing HIV-infected blood or, less frequently, after infected blood gets into a worker's open cut or a mucous membrane (for example, the eyes or inside of the nose). There has been only one instance of patients being infected by a healthcare worker in the United States – this involved HIV transmission from one infected dentist to six patients. Although people fear that HIV can be spread via other vectors, like mosquitoes, no such evidence exists. HIV is found in varying concentrations or amounts in blood, semen, vaginal fluid, breast milk, saliva, and tears. HIV does not survive well outside of the human body – you cannot get HIV from a toilet seat. Although HIV has been transmitted between family members in a household setting, this type of transmission is very rare. These transmissions are believed to have resulted from contact between skin or mucous membranes and infected blood. Casual contact through closed-mouth or "social" kissing is not a risk for transmission of HIV. It also appears that it is very difficult to contract HIV through "French" or open-mouth kissing, but the

CDC recommends against engaging in this activity with a person known to be infected. The CDC has investigated only one case of HIV infection that may be attributed to contact with blood during open-mouth kissing. HIV has been found in saliva and tears in very low quantities from some AIDS patients. It is important to understand that finding a small amount of HIV in a body fluid does not necessarily mean that HIV can be transmitted by that body fluid. HIV has not been recovered from the sweat of HIV-infected persons. Contact with saliva, tears, or sweat has never been shown to result in transmission of HIV.[142]

An estimated 2.8 million cases of chlamydia occur each year in the U.S. and more than 700,000 people are infected with gonorrhea annually. In addition, an estimated 45 million Americans over age 12 have been infected with herpes simplex virus – the primary cause of genital herpes. And as many as 20 million Americans are infected with human papillomavirus (HPV) – the virus that has been determined to cause cervical cancer. While syphilis rates have gone down over the past century and treatment has improved, syphilis is still around, especially in the urban South. There were 7,177 cases of syphilis reported to the CDC in 2004. Hepatitis B and C (viruses that infect the liver) can also be transmitted through sexual contact. Hepatitis B is a very common infection. Each year in the United States, an estimated 200,000 persons are newly infected with hepatitis B virus. More than 11,000 of these people are hospitalized, and 20,000 remain chronically infected. Overall, an estimated 1.25 million people in the United States have chronic hepatitis B virus infection, and 4,000 to 5,000 people die each year from liver disease or liver cancer related to hepatitis B. Hepatitis B virus is easily spread by direct contact with the blood or body fluids of an infected person. Hepatitis B can be transmitted from an infected mother to her baby at birth, through unprotected sex with an infected person, by sharing equipment for injecting street drugs, and by occupational contact with blood in a healthcare setting. People can have hepatitis B (and spread the disease) without knowing it. Sometimes, people who are infected with hepatitis B virus never recover fully from the infection. They carry the virus and can infect others for the rest of their lives. There is a vaccine for hepatitis B. Hepatitis C is responsible for 8,000 to 10,000 deaths per year in the U.S. The virus is spread through contact with infected blood and through sex. Most people don't know they carry the virus because they have either no symptoms or vague ones like fatigue. Only about 15% of those infected with HCV have a short-term infection that goes away by itself and never returns. The other 85% become chronically infected, meaning the virus stays in the liver, replicates, and may slowly attack the organ over a period of decades. Seventy percent of those infected with hepatitis C develop chronic liver disease, 15% develop cirrhosis over a period of 20-30 years, and 5% die from liver cancer or cirrhosis. Hepatitis C is the leading reason for liver transplantation in the United States. There is no vaccine for hepatitis C.[143] There are, however, several medications available now to treat Hepatitis C.

Emerging Infectious Diseases

While the known and common infectious agents cause the majority of illness in the U.S., there are several organisms that seem to grab the headlines because of their destructive potential. Such organisms are known as emerging infectious diseases, and are known as such because their rate has increased in the past two decades or threatens to increase in the near future. These emerging infectious diseases include: new infections resulting from changes or evolution of existing organisms; known infections spreading to new geographic areas or populations; previously unrecognized infections appearing in areas undergoing ecologic transformation; and old infections reemerging as a result of antimicrobial resistance in known agents or breakdowns in public health measures. Bird flu (avian influenza) is the current star of the emerging infection world. Bird flu has killed millions of birds (naturally or through intentional destruction) and around two hundred humans. The risk from avian influenza is generally low to most people, because the viruses do not usually infect humans. Most cases of avian influenza infection in humans have resulted from contact with infected poultry (e.g., domesticated chickens, ducks, and turkeys) or surfaces contaminated with secretion/excretions from infected birds. The spread of avian influenza viruses from one ill person to another has been reported very rarely, and transmission has not been observed to continue beyond one person. Unfortunately, however, more than half of those who have contracted the illness have died. There is not a vaccine for bird flu at present and the antiviral medicines that have been used to combat it seem to have limited effectiveness.[144]

Severe acute respiratory syndrome (SARS) was first identified in humans in early 2003. SARS typically begins with flu-like symptoms, including high fever that may be accompanied by headache and muscle aches, cough, and shortness of breath. Most people with SARS subsequently develop pneumonia. In the 2003 outbreak, there were more than 8,000 probable cases of SARS and 774 deaths (approximately 9% mortality) worldwide. Eight confirmed cases were identified in the United States. Of the 774 deaths attributed to SARS, more than 50% occurred in people 65 years of age or older. Susceptibility decreased significantly with age, with children the least likely to acquire the disease. The virus spreads primarily by close human contact. SARS-containing droplets can be released into the air when an infected person coughs or sneezes. Some specific medical procedures performed on SARS patients also can release virus-containing droplets into the air. Touching a SARS-infected surface and subsequently touching the eyes, nose, or mouth also may lead to infection. A SARS vaccine is currently being developed. The last case of SARS was reported in 2003, but health experts believe that it is possible for it to resurface.[145,146]

West Nile virus (WNV) made its first appearance in the United States in 1999. WNV is a flavivirus and it is spread by ticks and mosquitoes. Other well-known diseases caused by flaviviruses include yellow fever, Japanese encephalitis, dengue, and St. Louis encephalitis. People who contract WNV usually experience only mild symptoms – fever, headache, body aches, skin rash, and swollen lymph glands. If WNV enters the brain, however, it can cause life-threatening encephalitis (inflammation of the brain) or meningitis (inflammation of the lining of the brain and spinal cord). Most cases of disease occur in elderly people and those with impaired immune systems. Recent cases have shown that WNV can be transmitted through blood transfusions and organ transplants from WNV-infected donors. Health experts also believe it is possible for WNV to be transmitted from a mother to her unborn child and through breast milk. The first step in the transmission cycle of WNV occurs when a mosquito bites an infected bird or other infected animal. Crows are commonly associated with the virus because they are highly susceptible to infection. Scientists have identified more than 138 bird species that can be infected, and more than 43 mosquito species that can transmit WNV. Although the virus primarily cycles between mosquitoes and birds, infected female mosquitoes also can transmit WNV through their bites to humans and other "incidental hosts" such as horses. With so many susceptible hosts to amplify the virus and so many types of mosquitoes to transmit it, WNV has spread rapidly across the United States. WNV was first isolated in Uganda in 1937. Today it is most commonly found in Africa, West Asia, Europe, and the Middle East. In 1999, it was found in the Western Hemisphere for the first time in the New York City area. In early spring 2000, it appeared again in birds and mosquitoes and then spread to other parts of the Eastern United States. By 2004, the virus had been found in birds and mosquitoes in every state except Alaska and Hawaii. In 2005, WNV caused 2,949 cases of disease in the United States, including 116 deaths, according to the CDC. Human cases have now been reported throughout the continental United States, and in Canada and Mexico. A vaccine for WNV has been developed and is currently being tested.[147]

Multidrug-resistant tuberculosis (MDR-TB) is a form of tuberculosis that is resistant to two or more of the primary drugs used for the treatment of tuberculosis and it is another emerging disease. MDR-TB is already a huge problem in Third World countries especially where HIV is prevalent and has been a concern in the healthcare industry for many years – airborne transmission has been the cause of several well-publicized cases of nosocomial (hospital-based) outbreaks of MDR-TB in New York City and Florida. These outbreaks were responsible for the deaths of several patients and healthcare workers, a majority of whom were coinfected with HIV.[148] Resistance to one or several forms of treatment occurs when the bacteria develops the ability to withstand antibiotic attack and relay that ability to newly produced bacteria. In 2004, the CDC reported that 7.8% of tuberculosis cases in the U.S. were resistant to isoniazid, the first line drug used to treat TB. The CDC also reported that 1% of tuberculosis cases in the U.S. were resistant to both isoniazid and rifampin. Rifampin is the drug most commonly used with isoniazid. Overall, the number of MDR-TB cases were reported below 100 for the first time ever in 2003 but increased again to 101 in 2004. Only 27% of primary MDR-TB cases were in U.S. born persons. The percentage of U.S. born persons with MDR-TB has remained stable at approximately 0.6% since 2000. The proportion of MDR-TB cases among foreign-born persons has increased from 26% in 1993 to 73% of MDR-TB cases in 2004. The World Health Organization estimates that up to 50 million persons worldwide may be infected with drug resistant strains of TB. Also, 300,000 new cases of MDR-TB are diagnosed around the world each year and 79% of the MDR-TB cases now show resistance to three or more drugs.[149]

Mad Cow disease or BSE (bovine spongiform encephalopathy) is an emerging disease that has received a lot of attention lately. Mad Cow disease is a progressive neurological disorder of cattle that results from infection by an unusual transmissible agent called a prion. The nature of the transmissible agent is not well understood. Currently, the most accepted theory is that the agent is a modified form of a normal protein known as the prion protein. Research indicates that the first probable infections of BSE in cows occurred during the 1970s with two cases of BSE being identified in 1986. BSE possibly originated as a result of feeding cattle meat-and-bone meal that contained scrapie-infected sheep products. (Scrapie is a prion disease of sheep.) There is strong evidence and general agreement that the outbreak was then amplified and spread throughout the United Kingdom cattle industry by feeding rendered, prion-infected, bovine meat-and-bone meal to young calves. The BSE epidemic in the United Kingdom peaked in January 1993 at almost 1,000 new cases per week. Through the end of 2005 more than 184,000 cases of BSE had been confirmed in the United Kingdom alone in more than 35,000 herds. There exists strong epidemiologic and laboratory evidence for a causal association between a new human prion disease called variant Creutzfeldt-Jakob disease (vCJD) that was first reported from the United Kingdom in 1996 and the BSE outbreak in cattle. The interval between the most likely period for the initial extended exposure of the population to potentially BSE-contaminated food (1984-1986) and the onset of initial variant CJD cases (1994-1996) is consistent with known incubation periods for the human forms of prion disease. As of August of 2006, twelve cases of BSE had been identified in North America. Of these twelve cases, three were identified in the U.S. and nine in Canada. Four of the nine cases in Canada were born after the 1997 Canadian feed ban, and one was eight to ten years of age so may have been born before or just after the feed ban was implemented. Of the three cases identified in the U.S., one was imported from Canada. One of the cases identified in Canada was imported from the United Kingdom.[150,151]

And finally, Ebola is an emerging infectious disease that has many concerned due to its lethalness. Ebola is an often-fatal disease that affects humans and nonhuman primates (monkeys, gorillas, and chimpanzees), and it has appeared sporadically since its initial recognition in 1976. Ebola is believed to be a zoonotic (animal-borne) virus and is normally maintained in an animal host that is native to the African continent. The disease encompasses a range of symptoms, usually including vomiting, diarrhea, general body pain, internal and external bleeding, and fever. Mortality rates are generally high, ranging from 50% to 90%, with the cause of death usually due to shock or multiple organ failure. Confirmed cases of Ebola have been reported in the Democratic Republic of the Congo, Gabon, Sudan, the Ivory Coast, Uganda, and the Republic of the Congo. People can be exposed to Ebola virus from direct contact with the blood and/or secretions of an infected person. People can also be exposed to Ebola virus through contact with objects, such as needles, that have been contaminated with infected secretions. Ebola is especially dangerous in the healthcare setting because of its ability to spread rapidly.[152]

Where the Sick Get Sicker

Many urbanites head to hospitals and clinics when they are ill, but such facilities end up being a significant source of infectious disease. Healthcare-associated infections (HAIs) are infections that patients acquire during the course of receiving treatment for other conditions or that healthcare workers (HCWs) acquire while performing their duties within a healthcare setting. HAIs account for an estimated 2 million infections, 90,000 deaths, and $4.5 billion in excess healthcare costs annually. HAIs include infections of the urinary tract; surgical wounds; respiratory tract; skin (especially burns); blood; gastrointestinal tract; and central nervous system.

Methicillin-resistant *Staphylococcus aureus* (MRSA) is one such infection. Staph can cause infections that are resistant to treatment with usual antibiotics. Staph is commonly found on the skin and in the noses of healthy people. Occasionally, staph can cause infections; staph bacteria are one of the most common causes of skin infections in the United States. Most of these infections are minor (such as pimples, boils, and other skin conditions), and most can be treated without antimicrobial agents (also known as antibiotics or antibacterial agents). However, staph bacteria can also cause serious and sometimes fatal infections (such as bloodstream infections, surgical wound infections, and pneumonia). In the past, most serious staph bacterial infections were treated with a type of antimicrobial agent related to penicillin. Over the past 50 years, treatment of these infections has become more difficult because staph bacteria have become resistant to various antimicrobial agents, including the commonly used penicillin-related antibiotics. MRSA occurs most frequently among patients who undergo invasive medical procedures or who have weakened immune systems and are being treated in hospitals and healthcare facilities such as nursing homes and dialysis centers.

Chapter 6

The Case for the Other America

Adopt the pace of nature; her secret is patience.
~ Ralph Waldo Emerson

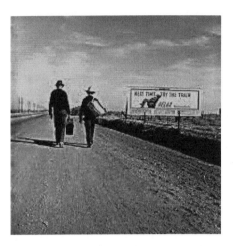

Leaving the City: The Case for the Other America

We hold these truths to be self-evident, that all men are created equal, that they are endowed by their Creator with certain unalienable Rights, that among these are Life, Liberty and the pursuit of Happiness.
~ *Declaration of Independence*

I have spent the preceding chapters identifying the threats to health and to some degree happiness one finds in big cities. The information I presented was pretty "thick" so I now will thin it out. Before I get into that though, let's start out at 35,000 feet and work our way down... literally. Take in the aerial pictures of cities, towns and rural communities taken at various heights below and then close your eyes and get a feeling for each one. Pretend you are a bird circling overhead looking for a place to land.

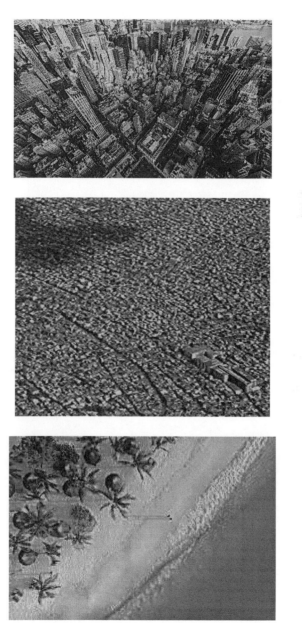

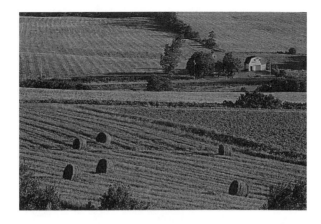

And now look at the following ground level pics and do the same visualization. This time you are a bird in the field or a city street.

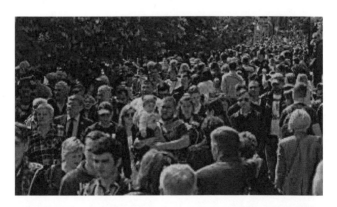

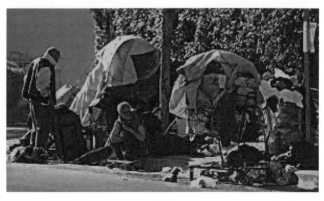

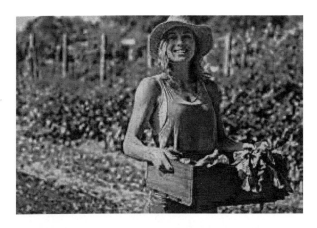

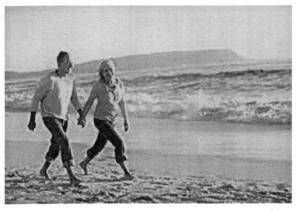

Which pictures appeal to you? If you answered A, B, E and/or F, then sorry – you might be an adrenaline junky. If you have a feeling of excitement from seeing tall buildings, crowds of people, and traffic... you might be addicted to stress. I get it. It's like an alcoholic passing a liquor store and then doubling back. But how does consuming crazy amounts of alcohol for long periods of time usually work out? Not good. Stress addiction is a killer. You may think it's making you stronger or smarter because you are surviving the chaos of the city, but you are really not. Chronic stress can wreak havoc on your mind and body. Your body is hard-wired to react to stress in ways meant to protect you against threats from predators and other aggressors. While we no longer have to worry about saber tooth tigers, that loud neighbor in apartment 210 and your ridiculous cable bill can get your cortisol and adrenaline pumping just the same. These constant hassles are perceived by your body as threats. Your hypothalamus, a region deep in your primitive brain, sets off an alarm system in your body. Through a combination of nerve and hormonal signals, this system prompts your adrenal glands, located atop your kidneys, to release a surge of hormones, including adrenaline and cortisol. Adrenaline increases your heart rate, elevates your blood pressure and boosts energy supplies. Cortisol, the primary stress hormone, increases sugars (glucose) in the bloodstream, enhances your brain's use of glucose and increases the availability of substances that repair tissues. Cortisol also curbs functions that would be nonessential or detrimental in a fight-or-flight situation. It alters immune system responses and suppresses the digestive system, the reproductive system and growth processes. This complex natural alarm system also communicates with the brain regions that control mood, motivation and fear. This cascade typically kicks in, lasts a few hours, then everything calms down. But if you become wired to see almost everything as a threat then your hypothalamus just keeps going. This is especially true of those who have had some trauma, PTSD. The long-term activation of the stress-response system and the overexposure to cortisol and other stress hormones that follows can disrupt almost all your body's processes. This puts you at increased risk of many health problems, including:

Anxiety
Depression
Digestive problems
Headaches
Heart disease

Sleep problems
Weight gain
Memory and concentration impairment
Cancer

We are all familiar with the scenario where let's say a man's wife of 50 years dies and it's not long until his death follows. Stress kills people. If you have a choice, and believe me you do, then why subject yourself to the daily onslaught of stressors one encounters in urban America? Urban life was tough before COVID and the civil disturbances, and now, well... it's pretty insane. Since COVID, when you see a crowd of people, do you think, "I wonder how many of them are infected with COVID?" If you see a field of cows, do you think, "I wonder how many of them are infected with COVID?" Of course not. According to the United Nations, 90% of reported COVID cases worldwide are concentrated in urban areas. That's certainly been the case here in the U.S. where major cities like New York, Chicago, Boston, Los Angeles, San Francisco, Houston, Dallas and Miami have been COVID-19 epicenters. Close your eyes again. Think about what kind of life you want. Where's your happy place?

As previously noted, roughly 80% of Americans live in urban areas, according to the U.S. Census Bureau. A recent Gallup poll, however, suggests many of them aren't happy living in the big city. Asked what kind of community they'd live in if they could move anywhere they wished, Americans overall said their number one choice would be in a rural area. Twenty-seven percent, specifically, said a rural area would be their ideal community, with an additional 12% opting for a small town. Just 12% said they'd prefer a big city, with an additional 21% preferring a big city suburb, the second-most-popular choice. Seventeen percent said a small city would be ideal, while just 10% said they'd like to live in a small city suburb.[153]

Happiness and well-being tend to be higher in rural areas than in urban ones. Urban areas also see higher rates of mental illness and poverty. Due to chronic underinvestment in infrastructure and housing, many cities have been doing a poor job of keeping pace with the flow of new arrivals, eroding the quality of life for everyone. Think about deteriorating Detroit or Milwaukee. Yes, urban life can be very good for those with high levels of education and financial resources, but it's not that great for those who work to service the wealthy. Depending on your level of income and education, an individual's urban experience may be accompanied by lower levels of social capital, higher levels of pollution, traffic congestion, crime, inequality, lack of green space, and exposure to diseases. While large cities constitute the driving force of developed economies and are still often seen as attractive places to live, their average levels of reported well-being show evidence of decline relative to rural environments when digital and other infrastructure develops in rural areas. If you can live wherever you want and have access to most of those things found in big cities, then evidence shows that people who live in rural areas are happier than their urban counterparts. If you're struggling to make ends meet to afford life in urban America, then maybe it makes more happiness and wallet sense to move to smaller America. Urban centers often develop the things one needs (like technology) to leave the urban center for other environments – this is known as the urban paradox, but once that happens then why stay if other living environs are ultimately more desirable. If you have children and you live in the city and are not wealthy, then raising them in the city makes little sense.

A recent study by the Vancouver School of Economics and McGill University looked at well-being at the level of more than 1,200 communities representing the country's entire geography. They were able to cross-reference the well-being responses with other survey data, as well as figures from the Canadian census, to see what sorts of characteristics were associated with happiness at the community level. Their chief finding is a striking association between population density – the concentration of people in a given area – and happiness. When the researchers ranked all 1,215 communities by average happiness, they found that average population density in the 20% most miserable communities was more than eight times greater than in the happiest 20% of communities. Their conclusion was that life was significantly less happy in urban areas. The authors found that the happiest communities had shorter commute times and less expensive housing. They also found that people in the happiest communities are less transient than in the least happy communities, that they are more likely to attend church and that they are significantly more likely to feel a sense of belonging in their communities. It's this sense of belonging that is a factor of major significance in community happiness studies.[154]

I understand that for many it's all about where the jobs are, but jobs often have to do with who you are. What kind of job do you want or need? And why do you want that job? Most people work to "earn a living." Yes, most people need money to live. Some people want to get rich, live the so-called American dream. Elon Musk is one such person. He's living the American dream. He can live anywhere he wants. In December of 2020, he essentially pulled the expensive Persian rug on the Bay Area and LA. He sold all of his real estate and moved his companies to Austin, burned-out on all the taxes and regulations of the less Golden State. Maybe he just wanted a breath of fresh air. Austin has a population density of 3,000 people per square mile; New York at 28,000; and San Francisco at 18,000. Or maybe he wanted more green… as in dollars. Texas has no state income tax; Californians can pay 11% or more. Oracle and Hewlett-Packard and, of course, their executives, left California soon after he did.

You don't have to be as rich as Elon Musk to pack up and leave. You don't even have to be that good at math. It's clear that living in smaller America is much cheaper than in most of America's big cities. There are many online cost of living calculators, but I'll use the one provided by NerdWallet here to make my case. Looking at some basic big city versus small city comparisons we see for someone who has an income of 100,000 the following expense differential:

	San Francisco	Dubuque, Iowa
2 Bedroom Apartment	4128 per mo	820 per mo
Median Home Price, 3 Br	1.2 million	285,000
Gasoline per gallon	4.82	2.76

	New York	Apple Valley, Ohio
2 Bedroom Apartment	5102 per mo	650 per mo
Median Home Price, 3 Br	2.2 million	235,000
Dozen eggs	2.25	1.25

	Los Angeles	Hannibal, MO
2 Bedroom Apartment	2850 per mo	825 per month
Median Home Price, 3 Br	859,676	135,000
Gasoline per gallon	4.70	2.39

Clearly, the cost of living is often substantially lower in smaller America mostly due to low housing costs. Now, add in a state that does not have income tax and things get even cheaper. Those states are: Alaska, Florida, Nevada, New Hampshire, South Dakota, Tennessee, Texas, Washington and Wyoming. And some states don't collect sales tax: Alaska, Delaware, Montana, New Hampshire, and Oregon. Sure, these lower cost of living places sometimes have wages that can be lower than the big city, but if you are working remotely with your big city salary then that doesn't matter much. One does have to keep in mind that sometimes one will have some different expenses moving from the city to the country, like buying a car and paying for gas, but the overall cost of living remains much lower. Whether you're a single young professional or just starting a family, conserving funds for the future should always be a high priority. If you are at or near retirement then best to stretch your retirement dollars. One of the best ways to free up and save income is to make sure you're in an area where the cost of living is reasonable... like the other America.

And, no, you won't be pulling up to a log cabin or a tent if you move to small town America. Let's use Muskogee, Oklahoma as an example. It ranks as one of the lowest cost of living cities in the U.S. Here's a nice house on nearly a half-acre for 152,000:

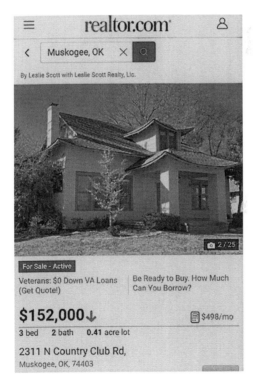

What can you buy in San Francisco for 150k? The monthly payment on such a home would be 500 per month with 30,000 down. The city of 37,000 is home to four institutions of higher learning, as well as the Oklahoma School for the Blind. The town also boasts six museums and the Oklahoma Music Hall of Fame. Major employers include the U.S. Department of Veterans Affairs, a VA medical center and paper company Georgia-Pacific. The unemployment rate in 2020 was 6%. And the average commute time is 12 minutes compared to 32 for LA. And, now let's get into that.

Commuting kills people. Long commutes are a fact of life in urban America. The average American commute time grew to just over 27 minutes one way in 2018, but people commuting hours a day in metro areas are not uncommon. The average American has added about two minutes to their one-way commute since 2009. That may not sound like a lot, but those numbers add up: the typical commuter now spends 20 more minutes a week commuting than they did a decade ago. The average round-trip commute time for New York City residents is now 81.6 minutes. The share of the population commuting there over two hours round-trip per day is 26.1%. Commuting exacts considerable stress on the human mind and body and on family relationships. Each added travel minute correlates with an increase in health problems. Several studies have shown that long-distance commuters suffer from psychosomatic disorders at a much higher rate than people with short trips to work. Physical symptoms range from headaches and backaches to digestive problems and high blood pressure. Mental ills include sleep disturbances, fatigue and concentration problems. And commuters get depressed. A recent study found that those with a commute of more than 90 minutes are far less likely to make trips for social purposes, such as to visit friends and relatives, play sports or go out to a movie. The divorce rate is much higher for long-distance commuters. Those who use public or mass transit often suffer the same fate, with the added bonus of being exposed to more infectious diseases. So why do individuals subject themselves and their families to this torture? There are three main reasons: a more interesting or better-paying job, the ability to own a home or live in a desirable area, and family priorities such as a better school or proximity to a partner's workplace. It may all start out as doable and worth it; people imagine they will long commute for a couple of years til the other job appears... but it rarely turns out that way.[155]

Unfortunately, life in the big city also became a whole lot more violent in 2020. Even if you are a staunch urbanite, you have to acknowledge things got bad and they were not off to a great start in 2021 – if you live in Washington DC then you live in a city that experienced a series of significant violent upheavals in 2020 that kept going in 2021. Civil disturbances or "riots," if you prefer that term, were ever present in 2020. Buildings were burned down, people fought, and police shot and were also beaten. Cities like Portland were in a state of perpetual disruption during 2020. In the fall of 2020, a report by the Council on Criminal Justice found homicides had increased sharply across 21 U.S. cities: Homicide rates increased by 42% during the summer and 34% in the fall over the summer and fall of 2019. Other data showed murder up 36% over 2020 in a sample of 51 U.S. cities. By the end of 2020, 1,066 people in the U.S. were killed by police. As of December 31, 2020, Chicago recorded 774 murders in 2020, an increase of more than 50% from the 506 murders in 2019. A real mess.

We are all familiar with the George Floyd-related protests and riots that lasted three weeks in June 2020 that covered 140 U.S. cities, including Minneapolis, Portland, Seattle, Washington DC, New York, Chicago, Philadelphia and Los Angeles. High-end boutiques in Beverly Hills and New York like Gucci and Chanel were looted, luxury stores in Santa Monica and big box retailers like Target and Macy's across the U.S. suffered tens of millions in losses. During that time, looters also struck at least 250 CVS pharmacies and 350 Walgreens nationwide. It is estimated that these disturbances will ultimately have direct costs of over 2 billion dollars. Thousands of businesses were lost, thousands of jobs lost, thousands of people injured. And just because that dust has settled somewhat, for now, that doesn't mean everything will go back to normal. Businesses near incident areas will continue to suffer lost revenues whether or not they incurred physical damage, mostly because people lose interest in or fear returning to areas impacted by the disturbances. It took areas of LA impacted by the Rodney King riots well over 10 years to get back to "normal."

And let's not forget about COVID's impact on urban America: over 35,000 dead in the New York metro area, over 25,000 dead in LA metro as of this writing. So many businesses shuttered, jobs lost and services discontinued. People locked down in their apartments. Children not in school. Since COVID-19, these trends and other preexisting inequities have been exacerbated and are reflected in deep declines in reported well-being. If you are a lower income urbanite, then recent well-being surveys show what would be predicted: poor people have much higher rates of worry, sadness, anger and loneliness relative to wealthier people. When it rains it pours.

As previously noted, social determinants of health are highly influential. The CDC defines social determinants of health as life-enhancing resources, such as food supply, housing, economic and social relationships, transportation, education, and healthcare, whose distribution across populations effectively determines length and quality of life. These include access to healthcare and resources such as food, insurance coverage, income, housing, and transportation.[156]

The World Health Organization has concluded that the unequal distribution of health-damaging experiences is not in any sense a "natural" phenomenon but is the result of a toxic combination of poor social policies, unfair economic arrangements – where the already well-off and healthy become even richer and the poor who are already more likely to be ill become even poorer – and bad politics. Living in environments where you at the mercy of others, politically or structurally, puts your health at risk.

The grass IS greener on the other side.

Tired of loneliness and alienation? How friendly are your neighbors? Do you even know who your neighbors are? How "involved" are people in your neighborhood or building? Not sure? No worries. The U.S. Senate's Joint Economic Committee Social Capital Project is a multi-year research effort that investigates the evolving nature, quality, and importance of our associational life. "Associational life" is shorthand for the web of social relationships through which people pursue joint endeavors – our families, our communities, our workplaces, and our religious congregations: "These institutions are critical to forming our character and capacities, providing us with meaning and purpose, and for addressing the many challenges we face." Robert Putnam, noted author of the book *Bowling Alone*, and the intellectual father of the concept of Social Capital, defines it as "social networks and the norms of reciprocity associated with them." The Brookings Institute further defines it:

Social capital involves relationships that are embedded within a group. Those relationships can have intrinsic value for the individual members, creating a sense of belonging or being connected to others. But it can also have value for the larger society for three reasons: first, because one can draw on it as a resource for accomplishing some objective, such as partnering with other parents to improve the local school; second, because it establishes or sustains certain values or norms of behavior such as being honest, tolerant, caring, and trusting of others; and third, because one's network may be a source of information, such as where the best jobs are.[157]

Social capital is a single score that's correlated with economic mobility, healthy families, widespread prosperity, and on the flip side, things like violent crime, opioid abuse, and digital addiction.

It essentially boils down to this: How cool are your neighbors? Can you borrow a cup of quinoa from them or what? The Joint Economic Committee has recently surveyed the country and have characterized states and counties on their levels of social capital. Nearly 60% of Americans reside in the bottom two-fifths of states for social capital. There is an unmistakable divide between North and South, with the bottom tier of states running in an unbroken stretch from Florida to California. New York is the only poorly ranked state that sits outside the South. New York City, however, does not fare well. Utah leads the nation in social capital alongside Minnesota and Wisconsin. The leading bloc runs through the mountain states up through the Dakotas and the Plains to the upper Midwest, while another centers on northern New England. It seems that wherever Mormons, Scandinavians, and Puritans settled you will likely find high levels of social capital. And, level of religious or church participation is not the driving factor. More than half of the metros with the highest social capital in America are in Minnesota, and the rest are in Utah, Iowa, and Wisconsin. All of the population centers in Maine, Vermont, and New Hampshire reside in the upper two-fifths of the ranking. On the other end of the index, there are just 10 counties across the Far South that rank well. Counties with large prisons or Native American reservations do particularly poorly.[158]

Recent studies have also shown that social capital indices are typically higher in rural versus urban environments. Rural communities consistently have higher levels of networks, civic participation and cohesion. Mental health indices score higher among rural residents. High population density is correlated with lower social capital.

And now a little more on the greener on the other side of the street. Ecopsychology is a growing field of study that looks at the relationship between being in nature and its impact on human health and happiness. Guess what? People who have some connection to the natural environment are healthier and happier people. In a study of 20,000 people, a team led by Mathew White, of the European Centre for Environment & Human Health at the University of Exeter, found that people who spent two hours a week in green spaces – local parks or other natural environments, either all at once or spaced over several visits – were substantially more likely to report good health and psychological well-being than those who don't. Study after study has shown that immersion in nature is critical to health, cognitive function and happiness. These studies have shown that time in nature is an antidote for stress. It can lower blood pressure and stress hormone levels, reduce nervous system arousal, enhance immune system function, increase self-esteem, reduce anxiety, and improve mood. Attention Deficit Disorder and aggression lessen in natural environments, which also help speed the rate of healing. In a recent study, psychiatric unit researchers found that being in nature reduced feelings of isolation, promoted calm, and lifted mood among patients. The growing body of research combined with an intuitive understanding that nature is vital and increased concerns about the exploding use of smart phones and other forms of technology has led to a tipping point at which health experts, researchers, and government officials are now proposing widespread changes aimed at bringing nature into people's everyday lives.[159] But, you don't have to wait for cities to figure out how to build more parks. You can just move to a more natural environment.

So, why do you live where you do? There are of course a variety of reasons with age and background figuring into the equation that determines where people live. Young people are often looking for excitement and so they often end up in cities. Older people are looking for peace so they end up in quiet towns. And families look for a house in the suburbs with a yard and good schools. Race, family and friends in the area, and gender also are factors. So is the "hometown" factor. North American Moving Services published a survey recently titled, "Why Americans Move?" They interviewed 2,000 Americans 25 years of age and older to understand why they live where they do. Nearly 72% of Americans live where they grew up. And women are more likely to stay near home: 75% of them stay near their hometown compared to 68% of men. People are also significantly influenced by housing costs. If you make 15 dollars per hour and local apartments cost 4,000 per month then you can't afford to live near work. So, if you like that job, then you are forced to commute. Many people have a vision that at some age they will settle in a single location and put down roots. Most people believe that this will happen for them between the ages of 24-26. A recent survey found that over 50% of people have lived in their current location for over 10 years, so people are very much creatures of habit.

Moving is not an easy thing, but every once and awhile there are mass migrations in the U.S., factors that force people to leave. During the 1930s roughly 2.5 million people left the Dust Bowl states – Texas, New Mexico, Colorado, Nebraska, Kansas and Oklahoma, due to years of drought. It was one of the largest migrations in American history. Oklahoma alone lost 440,000 people to migration. Many of them, poverty-stricken, traveled west looking for work. From 1935 to 1940, roughly 250,000 Oklahoma migrants moved to California. A third settled in the state's agriculturally rich San Joaquin Valley. These Dust Bowl refugees were called "Okies." Okies faced discrimination, menial labor and pitiable wages upon reaching California. Many of them lived in shanty towns and tents along irrigation ditches. "Okie" soon became a term of disdain used to refer to any poor Dust Bowl migrant, regardless of their state of origin.[160] It seems another mass migration, this time from urban America, has started.

COVID, the civil disturbances, and other factors inspired people to move in 2020. According to Cuebiq, a data firm that tracks movement via mobile phones, at one point in April 2020, Americans were relocating at twice the pace they did in 2019. Illinois, New York, and New Jersey are the three states with the most outbound moves. And people are moving out of California as well. The top inbound states in 2020 were Idaho, Arizona, Tennessee, South Carolina, Florida, Texas and North Carolina. One thousand people are moving to Florida every day. The most common reasons people move is a new job or the opportunity to move to their dream location. And some people will move for love too. But according to surveys, most need to know someone for at least two years to make a move of the heart as long as it doesn't raise their cost of living... no money, no honey.

So, where do you want to live? For the majority of people it truly is a choice. Many urbanites feel the city and its imagined possibilities will lead them to a better life, even after getting beat up by 2020. The job they have or the job they want to have is the end all. That thinking could instead lead them to the end of it all. As before, I can't tell you where to live. I have presented the case for life in the other America and in summary here are the principal reasons:

Cleaner Air

The further out of the city you get, the more the air quality improves. Polluted air damages your health, kills people.

Less Crime

Residents in rural areas are less likely to be the victims of a wide range of crimes versus those who are living in the city or suburbs. These include simple and aggravated assault, robbery, and theft.

Better Psychological Health

Living in an urban environment stimulates the brain in a negative way – fight or flight. Anxiety and depression rates are much higher in the big city.

Less Cost

Cities are more expensive to live in. Plain and simple.

Nature Benefit

Immersing yourself in a natural environment is good for everything from improving your short-term memory to lowering your blood pressure.

More Connection

The more people the harder it is to meet anyone. Big cities can be lonely places, small towns foster connection.

Community Spirit

People in small towns tend to be community-minded. There are lots of parades, festivals, and other gatherings and they are always looking for new faces.

Grow Your Own

Want to make use of those overalls and flannel shirts in the far reaches of your closet? If the Pilgrims figured out how to take care of themselves then so can you... and you have "How to" YouTube videos, they didn't.

Chapter 7

Further Thoughts and Resources

I would rather sit on a pumpkin, and have it all to myself, than be crowded on a velvet cushion.
~ Henry David Thoreau

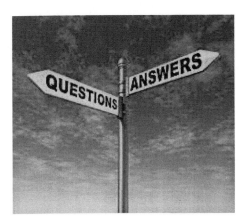

At this point in this book perhaps you are thinking, "Yep, that's it, I'm leaving the city." Or maybe you have already moved and you're thinking, "Seems like I made the right decision, urban living stinks," but you're still having some doubt. Moving, changing your life is obviously a big deal: not to be taken lightly no matter how good the argument is. We all make decisions, big and small, every day. How we arrive at those decisions varies from person to person. Some use their head, others use their gut, or their heart, or sometimes all three and more. There are many tools and guides to use to help you land on a decision. While it often seems like a simplistic exercise, it is often very helpful to put things down on paper. Use a pros and cons list to outline all of the advantages and disadvantages of a specific choice or decision. Consider what benefits, positive outcomes, and wins you anticipate as well as what costs, risks, or negative outcomes you might also anticipate. It's also a good idea to rank your entries or assign them points and add them up and find a winner.

Life changing decisions are rarely black and white, but you can get closer to making them more clear by asking yourself a series of questions. First, decide if your decision is something you want or something you need. Things you want are often influenced by others – wanting the same car your neighbor has. What one needs is deeply rooted in your values, ambitions, goals, and beliefs. Your path to self-actualization. Another way to look at this decision is how you will feel a year later if you don't do it. How much will you regret it? Also, don't think of the decision as the big thing; think of the goal as the big thing. Lay out what your life plan is and commit to it. If you don't know what your life plan is then spend more time meditating; the less you think the clearer things become. Don't fret the decision, dream of the ideal life for you. Write it down. Let's pretend you are told you have only six months left to live. How do you want to spend it? Use that as your guide.

While most decisions should come from your own heart, gut, head, it's not a bad idea to reach out to others for some advice. Some people have therapists, friends, and family to talk with to help them figure things out. One potential other source to use for guidance is a life coach. While "life coach" seems a little "California," many are quite good at getting you focused on figuring out what you want from life – getting you from point A to point B. Some life coaches specialize and focus on those who need help with decisions around moving. There are many paths for people to become a life coach, but some do have some legitimate training and certification. The International Coach Federation (ICF) is one body of certification. They define coaching as partnering with clients in a thought-provoking and creative process that inspires them to maximize their personal and professional potential. There are many life coach certifying bodies in the U.S., so it gets a bit confusing trying to figure out who is legit. A personal referral is often the best route here. Here are some resources to find a life coach that may be helpful:

https://www.tonyrobbins.com/coaching/find-life-coach-love/
www.expertise.com
www.bark.com
www.thumbtack.com

Comedian Jeff Foxworthy used to do a "Here's some signs you might be a redneck" routine that was a great way of highlighting that feature. So, I'm going to do something similar in a less comedic way: Here are some signs it might be time for you to leave the city:

- You are simply burned out – tired of everything in your city. Why have that kind of life?
- You need to be physically closer to your family and friends. Maybe you need them, maybe they need you. The circle of life.
- You want to change your line of work or job. Imagine your ideal job. If you can't do it where you live then move to where it's at.
- There's some place you've always wanted to live. There's no time like the present to be there. If you have visited a place and can't stop talking about how great it is then maybe you should live there.
- Your goals have changed. If you are no longer interested in a career in politics and live in DC, then maybe you shouldn't be there.
- You hate the weather. You hate rain and live in Seattle? Why?
- You've had a bad breakup and everything in your city reminds you of your ex.

- Someone you care about lives somewhere else. Nothing great about long-distance relationships. Now is maybe the time to shorten the distance.
- You're ready to start a family and the city you're in isn't the best place to raise children.
- Your favorite bar, restaurant, dog grooming salon has closed.
- You have no reason to stay.

If you are pretty settled on moving then here are some more things to consider as you move mentally closer to picking your ideal place to live:

- Don't move to a place where you don't know anyone. Maybe it sounds cool to completely blow things up, but it's so helpful to have a friend or two on the ground to help you get through the rough spots.
- Focus on the big things that bother you, not the small. Don't move to a new city to get away from a noisy neighbor, move to get away from a noisy city.
- Pick three things that make you extremely happy. Move to a place that has them.
- If you like to travel then pick a place with a decent and close airport.

All the Places You'll Go

If you are not sure where to move to then what follows is a very eclectic and pretty random selection of possibilities. Picking a new place to move to is definitely a heart, head, gut and perhaps a pelvis guided decision. It is, of course, worth the time, effort and money to visit the place you're considering moving to before you move there. Sure, there are many stories of people who went on a vacation to Hawaii and never left, but a lot of those stories are just stories. And be rational; if you hate the cold then don't consider moving to a cold place. Check in with the local Chamber of Commerce of the place where you're thinking of moving to get a sense of what is shaking there – https://www.uschamber.com/co/chambers.

So, pack your imaginary suitcase and here let's go on a little trek to find a place for you to move to.

You'd Have to Pay Me to Live There

There are a number of cities and towns across the country that will pay you to move there. No joke. And no, it's not because they are so awful, it's because they know that solid people help build up a community... the more you have the better it is for all. Some places also have a serious shortage of certain professionals – tech, healthcare, and that is the motivation. Tulsa, Oklahoma is offering a $10,000 relocation award along with a $1,000 housing stipend to move there. Tulsa has an extremely low cost of living. The oil-rich state of Oklahoma has a robust economy. Tulsa has a population of 400,000, a zoo, a museum and plenty of good eats. And if you get bored, you can use the 10,000 to go on a few vacations. What's not to like? Vermont is offering financial incentives that focus on remote workers. The Remote Worker Grant offers up to $10,000 in relocation expenses. The natural setting of Vermont appeals to anyone looking to escape an urban backdrop. Vermont is also a hub for craft beer, artisanal cheese and farmers' markets. It also has good skiing and Bernie... yes, Bernie. Are you a computer programmer? Then Chattanooga wants you. The city is looking to bolster its tech population. Their Geek Move program offers computer developers $1,250 in relocation expenses and a $10,000 forgivable mortgage. Chattanooga is listed as one of the top 20 cities for young homebuyers. If you love the great outdoors, then there is a lot to love in Tennessee. The Tennessee River and mountains are nearby for hiking, rock climbing, and kayaking. Downtown Chattanooga also offers lots of things to do, including a thriving arts scene, restaurants and shopping and family-friendly attractions like the Tennessee Aquarium and the River Pier. There are plenty of other states, cities and towns offering moving incentives. Is New York City offering any incentives? Forget about it.

Where Jesus Lives

Want to live in a place where the Bible is still bedside? A recently completed survey with 63,000 participants, conducted over the past 10 years, looked at rates of bible-mindedness (people who believe in the Bible) across America. As expected, the bible is still quite popular in the South, but not so much with people in the Northeast, Southwest, and West Coast. Twenty-seven percent of all Americans are bible-minded. The top five bible-minded cities are:

1. Birmingham, Alabama
2. Chattanooga, Tennessee
3. Tri-Cities, Tennessee
4. Roanoke, Virginia
5. Shreveport, Louisiana

There are very few bibles being thumped in New York, San Francisco and, of course, Las Vegas.

Where Jesus Isn't

The other end of the spectrum are places where people not only don't read the bible, they don't believe anything that's in it... atheists, agnostics, etc. Burlington, Vermont is one of the coldest cities in the United States, and it also has one of the largest atheist populations – seems the cold chases Jesus away. Boulder, Colorado has a large atheist population too. Boulder atheists posted billboards in 2012 calling God an "imaginary friend." New Hampshire is definitely secular and has several state representatives who self-identify as atheist. Further north in Portland, Maine, only 20% of the population identifies as religious. While the country was founded by religious-minded people, two of the places they settled, Massachusetts and Rhode Island, are two of the least religious states in the country.

Welcome to Paradise

Paradise, California is a town that seems to like (probably not) to burn down, and is the subject of the recent Ron Howard award-winning documentary, *Rebuilding Paradise*. It has a population of around 25,000 and it is located in Northern Cal on the way to Tahoe. Legend has it that the town was named because it was the home of the Pair o' Dice Saloon, an idea supported by a 1900 railroad map referring to the town as Paradice. In 2008, two wildfires nearly burned the town down. In 2019, the population was back up to around 5,000 as rebuilding continues. Maybe you can help to recreate the Paradise that was lost.

Can I Get an Oy Vey?

Like living among Jews? Most Jews live in or near big cities like New York, Boston, LA, and Miami. It is estimated that there are around 7 million Jews in the U.S. Around 8% of people in New York are Jewish. Most Jews live in areas where other Jews live. If you want a smaller, more suburban community of Jews then Kiryas Joel, near the Catskill Mountains in New York, may be the spot for you. The majority of the population are Yiddish-speaking, Hassidic Jews. In its favor, it's not an expensive place to live, but that's because incomes are so low. The village has the highest poverty rate in the nation. More than two-thirds of the residents live below the federal poverty line, and 40% receive food stamps.

Om Me

If Buddha is your thing, then there are plenty of places in the U.S. that are like-minded. While Buddhism is a mostly internally reflective practice, it is nice to connect with others who share the same knowledge, practices and beliefs. It is estimated that there are around three million practicing Buddhists in the U.S. Hawaii has the largest Buddhist population by percentage, amounting to 8% of the state's population. California follows Hawaii with 2%. Talmage, California, a town of 1,000 in Northern California, has the highest percentage of Buddhists per capita in the U.S. The community sits on 500 acres of land. It includes meadows, orchards, and forests and one of the first Buddhist monasteries built in the United States.

City of Ten Thousand Buddhas
http://www.cttbusa.org

Free Mantra Included

If you practice transcendental meditation then you probably know of Maharishi Vedic City (MVC), a city in Jefferson County, Iowa. It has a population of around 1,300 and is approximately one square mile. The goals of the community are to "protect, nourish, and satisfy everyone, upholding the different social, cultural, and religious traditions while maintaining the integrity and progress of the city as a whole." That's cool. It also has a university, the Maharishi University of Management.

https://maharishivediccity-iowa.gov

Hell Is Not As Hot As You Think

Hell, Michigan is an unincorporated community in Livingston County in the U.S. state of Michigan. As an unincorporated community, Hell has no defined boundaries or population statistics of its own. It is located within Putnam Township. Hell developed around a sawmill, gristmill, distillery and tavern. All four were operated by George Reeves, who moved to the area in the 1830s from the Catskill Mountains in New York. He purchased a sawmill on what is now known as Hell Creek in 1841. In addition to the sawmill, Reeves purchased 1,000 acres surrounding the mill. Reeves then built a gristmill on Hell

Creek which was powered by water that was impounded by a small dam across the creek. Farmers in the area were quite successful in growing wheat and had an abundance of grain. Reeves opened a distillery to process the excess grain into whiskey. Reeves also opened a general store and tavern on his property. There are a number of theories for the origin of Hell's name. The first is that a pair of German travelers stepped out of a stagecoach one sunny afternoon in the 1830s, and one said to the other, "So schön hell!" ("So beautifully bright!") Their comments were overheard by some locals and the name stuck. Another story is that soon after Michigan gained statehood, George Reeves was asked what he thought the town he helped settle should be called and replied, "I don't care. You can name it Hell for all I care." The name became official in 1851.

Disneyland Is Not the Happiest Place On Earth

What makes a happy city? Is it the climate? Is it the people or the variety of things to do? How about the great jobs? WalletHub recently conducted their annual study of the happiest cities in the U.S. and listed below are their findings. Their rankings are based on 30 key indicators of happiness, ranging from depression rate to income-growth rate to average leisure time spent per day. Here is their top ten:

1. Fremont, CA
2. Plano, TX
3. San Jose, CA
4. Irvine, CA
5. Madison, WI
6. Sioux Falls, SD
7. Huntington Beach, CA
8. Scottsdale, AZ
9. Santa Rosa, CA
10. Pearl City, HI

LA came in at number 80; New York at 86; and Chicago at 113. Not surprising.[161]

https://wallethub.com/edu/happiest-places-to-live/32619

Men's Health did their ranking of happiest cities in 2020. Their in-depth research looked at well-being, mental health, community engagement, financial well-being, access to environment and physical health. Here are their rankings:

1. Lincoln, NE
2. Madison, WI
3. Raleigh, NC
4. Portland, ME
5. Billings, MT
6. Sioux Falls, SD
7. Burlington, VT
8. Minneapolis, MN
9. Anchorage, AK
10. Denver, CO

Other surveys have looked at happy smaller towns and cities and here's some of the ones often highlighted in such surveys:

Charlottesville, Virginia

Nicknamed Joy Town, USA, this historic place offers a sense of community, higher education (the University of Virginia) and other amenities usually reserved for larger cities.

Southport, North Carolina

Residents of this tiny 2.2-square-mile harbor town almost exclusively walk, bike or drive golf carts to get from place to place. This, paired with tons of Southern charm and pristine views, makes it an idyllic place to live.

Los Alamos, New Mexico

Los Alamos shows up on many "great place to live" lists and it's growing as a result. It is nestled in the Rio Grande River Valley, surrounded by the Jemez Mountains. There's a diverse and super-involved community there and an extremely educated population. It has a rich history related to the development of the atomic bomb at Los Alamos Laboratory.

Stillwater, Oklahoma

The commute time is close to nothing, the cost of living and unemployment very low in this Midwestern college town – the home of Oklahoma State University. The residents there have low stress rates and an endless supply of things to do.

State College, Pennsylvania

The town is located in what's known as "Happy Valley." It is, of course, the home of Penn State. It's one of the most walkable places in the country, it has an average commute time well below average and most residents own their own homes.

Delray Beach, Florida

Known as Florida's "Village by the Sea," this community doesn't feature a single high rise building so water views are by the plenty. And the white sand public beaches are simply magnificent. Delray's Atlantic Avenue is one of the most happening streets in the U.S.

Wellfleet, Massachusetts

This Cape Cod-based town is famous for its mild, sweet oysters. This small town has nine beaches, white-clapboard New England-style homes and a trendy restaurant scene.

Get Down (the Hill)

If skiing is your thing then why not move to a place where you can do it often? Can you imagine how good of a skier, and how in shape, you'd be if you skied 100 days per year? Here, according to SmartAsset, are the best ski towns to live in America:

Jackson, Wyoming

Wyoming's Jackson Hole Ski Resort offers some of the best skiing not only in the country but in the world, and is one of the nation's premier destinations for winter sports. Unlike many ski town economies, commercial activity in Jackson does not wane in the summer. Because of its proximity to Grand Teton National Park and Yellowstone National Park, tourism is a year-round industry in Jackson.

Hailey, Idaho

Located in the Sun Valley region of Idaho, Hailey is near the world-famous Sun Valley ski resort. The area is a year-round draw for outdoor enthusiasts, with the surrounding Sawtooth National Forest offering superb hiking and fishing throughout the summer.

Snoqualmie, Washington

Twenty-five miles down I-90 from The Summit at Snoqualmie ski area, Snoqualmie, Washington may be the only town on this list in which snow is a rarity. Even when blizzard conditions are in effect at the Summit, it is often cool and rainy in Snoqualmie the town (which sits at a significantly lower altitude than the ski area). For those who want a high quality of life near great skiing, however, the Snoqualmie Valley may be the perfect choice. Snoqualmie enjoys the lowest violent crime rate of any town we examined, and the sixth highest disposable income.

June Lake, California

Located a half hour north of Mammoth Mountain, June Lake is Mammoth's chill cousin with around 700 year-round residents. June may be small – just 1,500 skiable acres and seven lifts, but has some of the best backcountry skiing in the U.S. June is starting to get a lot of developer notice, so get there before it is less chill.

These are just a few of the awesome ski towns you can call home. Just need to pack up your skis and move there.[162]

No Dummies Please

Not that graduating from college makes you smart or interesting, but some people have a preference to live around other college grads – I guess so they can argue about who has the best football team. WalletHub put together a list of cities with high percentages of college grads, but quality of local schools also factored in their rankings.

Ann Arbor, Michigan

Ann Arbor, the hometown of the University of Michigan, a top-notch university, had the highest percentage of bachelor's degree holders per capita in their study. It also has a very high percentage of residents with professional and graduate degrees.

Alexandria, Virginia

Sixty-one percent of the 100,000 plus Alexandria residents have at least a bachelor's degree. Alexandria is also home to Virginia Theological Seminary and satellite campuses of Virginia Tech, Virginia Commonwealth University, and George Washington University. It is home to numerous government agencies and private corporations.

Arlington, Virginia

Arlington is another brainy city. Consistently ranked among the most affluent, educated, and forward-thinking DC suburbs, the city has 18 colleges of higher learning including Marymount University, George Mason University, Virginia Tech, DeVry University, and Strayer University as well as a myriad of technical and professional schools and institutes.

Boulder, Colorado

The home of CU Boulder maintains an estimated 192,815 people over age 25, 58.3% of which hold a bachelor's degree or higher. It is home to the Culinary School of the Rockies and 11 research institutes. Whole Foods has their headquarters there.

Cambridge, Massachusetts

Cambridge is home to 10 colleges and universities, including the American Academy of Arts and Sciences, Harvard University and MIT. Biotechnology firms dominate the private sector in the area, with companies such as GlaxoSmithKline, AstraZeneca, Shire, and Pfizer in the mix.

There are, of course, other brainy areas of the country – Bay Area and Seattle, but the ones noted above win out when it comes to percent of population with bachelor degrees or higher.

Nerd Alert: Miami is the fastest growing recent college grad city in the U.S.

Where Did Everyone Go?

A lot of people moved during 2020, around one-fifth of people in the U.S. ... double the amount in 2019. Most people headed West and South in 2020, with Idaho experiencing the most inbound moves and New Jersey seeing the most outbound moves, according to data from several moving companies. And yes, many moved due to the pandemic. Idaho had the highest percentage of inbound migration at 70%, with more people saying they moved there for cost-of-living reasons than any other state. Here's a little intel on three of the hottest move cities.

Boise, Idaho

The capital of Idaho has been experiencing big growth in its population and its home values in recent years. From 2010 to 2020, Boise's population rose by about 12%, from 209,578 people to 234,576. From October 2015 to October 2020, home values rose by 75% on average, with the value of a typical home in Boise up to $379,161 from $216,607 five years ago.

Killeen, Texas

Since 2010, Killeen's population has grown by about 20%, from 128,980 people to 153,973 in 2020. Home values have steadily increased in Killeen, and the pace of sales is cranking up. Last year, there were 1,186 homes available for sale in the Killeen metro area in October 2019. In October 2020 the inventory was down to just 450 homes. How do you like them doggies?

Spokane, Washington

Is located in Spokane and they have been the NCAA's hottest basketball team over the past few years. And now Spokane's real estate market is matching the Zag's heat. Spokane home values have grown robustly lately, with the value of a typical home rising by 14.4% in just one year, from $249,055 in October 2019, up to $284,800 in October 2020. Homes in the Spokane metro area are selling quickly. In October 2020, more than two-thirds of homes sold were taken off the market within two weeks.

In addition to the above noted cities, Tampa, Jacksonville, and of course, Austin, have been growing and continue to grow like crazy. Austin has added 200,000 people in the last 10 years – up 25%. New York City is up 2% in the past 10... you starting to get a sense of what's happening?

Beach Me

Living by the ocean is almost always good, but some beach towns are definitely better than others. Most of us have vacationed at the beach and had those "I don't want to leave" moments. Here's a few beach towns that are always on critics' best list:

Nags Head, North Carolina

Nags Head is the name for a trio of beach towns in the Outer Banks. Nags Head proper stretches for 11 miles of beach and sound, which includes the tallest sand dune on the East Coast. Nags Head is rich in aviation history with the Wright Brothers doing most of their flight tests there back in the day. It's also a mecca for East Coast surfers.

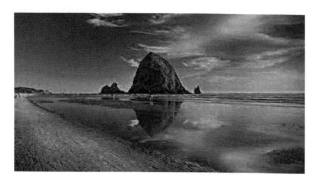

Cannon Beach, Oregon

Cannon Beach is home to Oregon's famed Haystack Rock. That sight alone should be enough to keep you engaged for a long time, but little Cannon also has dog beaches, restaurants, breweries, and many galleries. Take a visit and you won't want to leave.

Tybee Island, Georgia

Tybee is 30 minutes from Savannah at the easternmost point of Georgia. It's an island of wide, sandy beaches with a laid-back vibe. It's colorful and full of history… and Southern charm.

Santa Barbara, California

It doesn't get much better than Santa Barbara. It's the best of Spain-flavored California; it's mountains and beaches. It's rural wineries and some downtown urban funk. It's a college town that is also home to some of the richest and most famous people in the U.S… rhymes with Oprah.

Paia, Maui, Hawaii

That's right folks, Hawaii is part of the U.S. Paia is an awesome Hawaiian surf town – it's free of big resorts and all… funky chill with a population of 2,500. It's also one of the best windsurfing spots in the world.

I Like it Red

We have spent the last 10 years talking about red states and blue states. You know where they are and you know what you are. I'm not going to spend much time on this, but to say, if you want it conservative then Midland, Texas might be your spot. Midland has not voted for a Democrat for president since Harry Truman in 1948.

I Like it Blue

Most big cities in the United States rate as "liberal." In 2020, we got a better sense of how truly "blue" some cities are – Portland, Seattle, Minneapolis. Berkeley has long been considered to be the most liberal city in America and probably still is, but if you like "ice blue," then let me introduce you to Fargo. North Dakota has traditionally been a conservative state while Fargo tends to be the most liberal area of the state. In 2008 Obama won Cass County, where Fargo is located, but lost the rest of the state. So, if you loved the movie and you're liberal, put on your thickest jacket and give Fargo a spin.

I Like it Green

Are you rich? Or do you like being around rich people? Or both? Here are some not so obvious, more out of the way places that are money:

Williston, North Dakota

The city of Williston expanded rapidly during the first half of the 2010s, driven by the explosion in shale oil drilling that once gave North Dakota the fastest-growing economy in the nation. If you want rich neighbors, but hate the cold and fracking, then this isn't your place.

Torrington, Connecticut

Torrington has long been a popular retreat for Manhattan's wealthy and chic looking for a remote, mountainous retreat. It's also home for many of Connecticut's homegrown millionaires.

Juneau, Alaska

Because of its remote location, everything is a bit pricier in Juneau. Groceries alone cost almost 40% more than the U.S. national average. On the plus side, Alaska is one of the most tax-friendly states in the union. Not only is there no state income tax, but the government actually pays residents an annual stipend. Most of Juneau's millionaires are oil rich.

Summit Park, Utah

Skiing, luxury shopping, world famous film festivals – the Summit Park, Utah, area has everything a millionaire could ask for and more. The Summit Park micro area, which also includes Park City, is a short drive from Salt Lake City and has the second highest concentration of millionaire households of any small town in the U.S. Lots of great skiing there and the annual Sundance film festival.

Los Alamos, New Mexico

Los Alamos has a very high concentration of millionaire households, not the total number of millionaires. And on that relative basis, Los Alamos really stands out. It's also a "smart" town with a very high percentage of the population with advanced degrees.

I Like the Other Green

You like farmers' markets and eating organic? Well, then the West is pretty deep green. Most surveys focused on healthy eating cities usually put Portland, San Francisco, and Seattle at the top. Colorado is also pretty "crunchy." If you like your organic salad mixed with politics then Washington DC is the place for you.

Grow Your Own

If you are contemplating moving to a place where you can have your own little (or big) farm then there are some states that are more favorable than others for that purpose. Yes, you can grow fruits and vegetables in every state in the U.S., but Wyoming's produce is no match for California's. Every state has their thing, but some people grow year round in their basements and make some good money doing so – it's not unusual to net over 50,000 per year if done right. California rarely freezes so is great for most crops. It's the cost of land there and the bureaucracy that kills things. Iowa is big on produce, but also big on winter freezes. The land, however, is plentiful and cheap; you just have to pick the right crops. Indiana, Missouri, Kansas and Nebraska are also great for farms big and small. Vermont has a very high percentage of farmers, and lots of farmers' markets. People in Vermont are dedicated to purchasing locally-sourced food, so hobby farmers can do quite well. Farming and ranching have always been big in Texas, and there is still plenty of good land available for purchase. Hay, wheat, soybeans, cotton and corn are common crops grown in the Lone Star state. Livestock choices include the classic cattle, horses, goats, sheep and pigs. If you prefer more exotic livestock, there are also plenty of emu farmers and people raising bison as well.

Okay, Just One

There are so many Best Places to Live lists. It makes little sense to post them because they are easily found on the Internet, but here's the top five from Livability for 2020. They surveyed over a thousand people and used a variety of other data to form their list. Their main themes were affordability, job opportunities, diversity and inclusion.

1. Fort Collins, CO
   Population: 170,243
   Set against the foothills of the Rocky Mountains, Fort Collins is a vibrant and growing city that's overflowing with opportunity. It's home to Colorado State University.
2. Ann Arbor, MI
   Population: 119,980
   Ann Arbor also shows up on many "brainiest" places list as previously discussed.
3. Madison, WI
   Population: 259,680
   Madison is full of everything. Another vibrant college town that often shows up on other "best" lists.
4. Portland, ME
   Population: 66,215
   Portland has a supportive business climate, incredible quality of life and creative residents.
5. Rochester, MN
   Population: 118,935
   Home of the Mayo Clinic and so much more. Minnesota often tops the best public schools in the U.S.

As you can see above, LA, NYC and Chicago not on the list.[163]

Getting Your Move On

As we have discussed, moving is a big deal. It's emotionally and physically exhausting, costly, stressful, time consuming... an overall major pain. But, when you settle into your new place it won't take all that long to get a smile back on your face. Regardless of the reason, moving represents one thing – chance at a happier life.

Many people struggle with whether or not to hire a moving company when they decide to move. Moving a two-bedroom house across the country will cost around 10,000. The cost of a cross-country U-Haul is at least 3,000. So, there you have it. It will cost you around 7,000 dollars to lift 20,000 dollars of stress and headache. Another approach is to downsize big time and load up your car. Go through all of your stuff and absolutely get rid of clothes and things you don't use. Do a closet purge. If it doesn't fit, is out of style, and/or you haven't worn it in a year, get rid of it. Get rid of items you wouldn't buy again. When deciding whether an item serves a purpose in your life ask yourself whether you would go out and spend money on it if you didn't already have it. If you wouldn't, you likely don't need it. Take a picture for memory sake, and donate or trash it. And then drive your lightly-stuffed car or truck to your new home.

There are plenty of moving calculators for you to try to get a better sense of cost of the move if you don't want to downsize.

Here's one from moving.com:

https://www.moving.com/movers/moving-cost-calculator.asp

The folks at move.org have put together reviews of moving companies if you want to go that route:

https://www.move.org/best-interstate-moving-companies/

Relocation Services

He who hires themself as a relocation specialist has a fool for a client.

Sure, you're smart. You have the Internet and can figure everything out. You know, however, that doesn't always work. Sometimes you need to connect with people, and in the case of moving you need to talk to a lot of people. Some of the people you should talk to are relocation specialists. The majority of them work out of or with realty offices, some work on the corporate side of things. A relocation specialist is an expert who manages the details involved with relocating to a new area. These specialists work nationwide and sometimes worldwide, to make moving as painless as possible. Some relocation specialists get paid by referral fees from the vendors and moving companies they work with, rather than charging their clients directly. If you are buying a new home, they will also help you with some of the work that relates to your new home. If contractors are doing work on your new home before you arrive, your relocation service can be there to supervise. Here are some highly rated companies for you to connect with:

HomeServices Relocation
www.homeservicesrelocation.com

Corporate Relocation International
corprelo.com

Signature Relocation
www.signaturerelo.com

TRC Global Mobility, Inc.
www.trcglobalmobility.com

Seek out a real estate agent in the area you are considering who is a relocation expert. There are so many great real estate-related websites these days with so much info beyond the typical house-hunting queries like crime and other neighborhood related data. Here are the popular sites:

www.realtor.com
www.zillow.com
www.redfin.com
www.trulia.com
www.homes.com

These sites are also useful for those interested in renting instead of buying.

In conclusion, not that anything ever concludes, if you are not happy with where you live then think about or plan on moving. Change, while often scary, can bring so much good if it is change for a well purposed reason. For many, life in the big city is akin to an abusive relationship. You know it's wrong, but you can't seem to get out of it. It becomes easier once you admit it's a problem. Enlist the support of others. Stop making excuses for your city. Seek help from others. Visit more desirable places and see what it feels like to be there. And, don't worry that your city will fall apart if you leave. It won't even miss you.

Endnotes

1. Odds of Dying. 2020, June 22. Retrieved January 03, 2021, from https://injuryfacts.nsc.org/all-injuries/preventable-death-overview/odds-of-dying/

2. Conover, C. 2020, October 21. What Is Your Risk Of Dying From Covid-19? Retrieved January 03, 2021, from https://www.forbes.com/sites/theapothecary/2020/10/06/what-is-your-risk-of-dying-from-covid-19/?sh=719f415d6159

3. Centers for Disease Control and Prevention. Life Expectancy. http://www.cdc.gov/nchs/fastats/lifexpec.htm (accessed 30 October 2006).

4. Kaplan, H., K. Hill, J. Lancaster, and A.M. Hurtado. 2000. A Theory of Human Life History Evolution: Diet, Intelligence, and Longevity. *Evolutionary Anthropology* 9 (4): 156-185.

5. Diener, E., E.M. Suh, R.E. Lucas, and H.E. Smith. 1999. Subjective Well-Being: Three Decades of Progress. *Psychological Bulletin* 125: 276-302.

6. Maslow, Abraham. 1962. *Toward a Psychology of Being*. New York: Van Nostrand.

7. Clayman, Charles. 2004. *The American Medical Association Family Medical Guide, 4th Edition*. Wiley.

8. Maslow, A.H. 1965. A Theory of Human Motivation. *Psychological Review* 50, 370-396.

9. Mumford, Lewis. 1938. *The Culture of Cities*. New York: Harcourt, Brace and Co.

10. Toynbee, Arnold. 1967. *Cities of Destiny*. New York: McGraw-Hill.

11. Gottmann, Jean. 1961. *Megalopolis: The Urbanized Northeastern Seaboard of the United States*. New York: The Twentieth Century Fund.

12. Chandler, Tertius. 1987. *Four Thousand Years of Urban*

Growth: An Historical Census. St. David's University Press.

13. Gibbon, Edward. 1906. *The History of the Decline and Fall of the Roman Empire*. New York: Fred de Fau and Co.

14. Chandler, Tertius. 1987. *Four Thousand Years of Urban Growth: An Historical Census*.

15. Frey, William and Speare, Alden. 1988. *Regional and Metropolitan Growth and Decline in the United States*. New York: Russell Sage Foundation.

16. U.S. Census Bureau, Census History Staff. Urban and Rural Areas. www.census.gov. Retrieved 2019-01-08.

17. U.S. Census Bureau. 2020. The U.S. Census. https://www. census.gov/data/tables/time-series/demo/popest/2010s-total-cities-and-towns.html (accessed 07 December 2020).

18. National Association of County and City Health Officials. 2003. Big Cities Health Inventory. http://www.naccho. org/pubs/product1.cfm?Product_ID=101 (accessed 29 October 2006).

19. Milgram, Stanley. 1970. The Experience of Living in Cities. *Science* 167:1461-1468.

20. Regoeczi, Wendy C. 2002. The Impact of Density: The Importance of Nonlinearity and Selection on Flight and Fight Response. *Social Forces* 81: 505-530.

21. Christenfeld, Nicholas et al. 1999. Exposure to New York City as a Risk Factor for Heart Attack Mortality. *Psychosomatic Medicine* 61:740-743.

22. World Health Organization. 2006. Millennium Ecosystem Assessment. http://www.millenniumassessment.org/en/ index.aspx (accessed 10 October 2006).

23. The Paris Agreement. (n.d.). Retrieved January 03, 2021, from https://unfccc.int/process-and-meetings/the-paris-agreement/the-paris-agreement

24. Mokdad, A., J.S. Marks, D.F. Stroup, and J.L. Gerberding. 2004. Actual Causes of Death in the United States, 2000. *JAMA* 291:1238-1245.

25. World Health Organization (WHO). 2004. Children's Environmental Health. http://www.who.int/ceh/publications/atlas/en/ (accessed 10 October 2006).

26. Environmental Protection Agency (EPA). 2006. Air Now. http://airnow.gov/ (accessed 10 October 2006).

27. EPA. 2006. Plain English Guide to the Clean Air Act. http://www.epa.gov/air/oaqps/peg_caa/pegcaa04.html (accessed 10 October 2006).

28. American Lung Association State of the Air. 2021. State of the Air | American Lung Association. (n.d.). Retrieved October 15, 2021, from https://www.lung.org/research/sota

29. The Met Office. 2006. The Great Smog of 1952. http://www.metoffice.com/education/secondary/students/smog.html (accessed 10 October 2006).

30. Dhara, V. and R. Dhara. 2002. The Union Carbide Disaster in Bhopal: A Review of Health Effects. *Archives of Environmental Health* 57(5):391-404.

31. Health impact of pollution: State of the Air. Health Impact of Pollution | State of the Air | American Lung Association. (n.d.). Retrieved October 15, 2021, from https://www.lung.org/research/sota/health-risks

32. Tobacco Health Effects. 2020, April 28. Retrieved January 03, 2021, from https://www.cdc.gov/tobacco/basic_information/health_effects/index.htm

33. What is California's wildfire smoke doing to our health? Scientists paint a bleak picture. 2020, September 04. Retrieved January 03, 2021, from https://www.theguardian.com/world/2020/sep/04/what-is-californias-wildfire-smoke-doing-to-our-health-scientists-paint-a-bleak-picture

34. Churg, A., M. Brauer, T.I. Fortoul, and J.L. Wright et al. 2003. Chronic exposure to high levels of particulate air pollution and small airway remodeling. *Environ Health Perspect.* 111: 714-718.

35. Gauderman, W.J., G.F. Gilliland, H. Vora et al. 2002. Association between air pollution and lung function growth in southern California children: Results from a second cohort. *Am J Respir Crit Care Med.* 166:76-84.

36. Ibid.

37. Lin, S., J.P. Munsie, S-A Hwang, E. Fitzgerald, and M.R. Cayo. 2002. Childhood Asthma Hospitalization and Residential Exposure to State Route Traffic. *Environ Res.* 88:73-81.

38. American Lung Association. Ozone. https://www.lung. org/clean-air/outdoors/what-makes-air-unhealthy/ozone (accessed 10 October 2021).

39. Bell, M.L., A. McDermott, S.L. Zeger, J.M. Samet, and F. Dominici. 2004. Ozone and Short-term Mortality in 95 US Urban Communities. *JAMA* 292:2372-2378.

40. EPA. 2006. About Air Toxics. http://www.epa.gov/ttn/ atw/allabout.html (accessed 15 October 2006).

41. Health impact of pollution: State of the Air. Health Impact of Pollution | State of the Air | American Lung Association. (n.d.). Retrieved October 15, 2021, from https://www.lung.org/research/sota/health-risks

42. EPA. 2006. Indoor Air Quality. http://www.epa.gov/iaq/ ia_faqs.html (accessed 15 October 2006).

43. Building Science Corporation. 2002. What Relative Humidity Should I Have in My House? www.buildingscie nce.com/resources/moisture/relative_humidity_0402.pdf (accessed 15 October 2006).

44. EPA. 2006. Indoor Air Quality. http://www.epa.gov/iaq/ ia_faqs.html (accessed 15 October 2006).

45. EPA. 2006. Radon. http://www.epa.gov/radon/ (accessed 15 October 2006).

46. Environmental Protection Agency. (n.d.). EPA. Retrieved October 15, 2021, from https://www.epa.gov/indoor- airquality-iaq/formaldehydes-impact-indoor-air-quality

47. EPA. 2021. Volatile Organic Compounds. http://www. epa.gov/iaq/voc.html (accessed 15 October 2021).

48. EPA. 2021. Carbon Monoxide. http://www.epa.gov/iaq/ co.html (accessed 15 October 2021).

49. EPA. 2021. Nitrogen Dioxide. http://www.epa.gov/iaq/ no2.html (accessed 15 October 2021).

50. NIOSH. 2021. Drycleaning. http://www.cdc.gov/niosh/ topics/dryclean/ (accessed 15 October 2021).

51. EPA. 2021. Lead. http://www.epa.gov/iaq/lead.html (accessed 15 October 2021).

52. Exide lead contamination. 2020, December 08. Retrieved January 03, 2021, from https://en.wikipedia.org/wiki/ Exide_lead_contamination

53. EPA. 2021. Pesticides. http://www.epa.gov/iaq/pesticid. html (accessed 15 October 2021).

54. EPA. 2021. Asbestos. www.epa.gov/asbestos (accessed 15 October 2021).

55. EPA. 2021. Mold. http://www.epa.gov/mold/ (accessed 15 October 2021).

56. EPA. 2021. Sick Building Syndrome. http://www.epa.gov/ iaq/pubs/sbs.html (accessed 10 October 2021).

57. WHO. 2006. Water Sanitation and Health. http://www. who.int/water_sanitation_health/en/ (accessed 20 October 2006).

58. Viessman, W. and M.J. Hammer. 2005. *Water Supply and Pollution Control*. Upper Saddle River, NJ: Prentice Hall.

59. EPA. 2006. Water. http://www.epa.gov/ow/ (accessed 10 October 2006).

60. NRDC. 2005. Bottled Water: Pure Drink or Pure Hype? http://www.nrdc.org/water/drinking/bw (accessed 20 October 2006).

61. MMWR. (n.d.) Hurricanes. http://www.cdc.gov/mmwr/ mguide_nd.html (accessed 20 October 2006).

62. USGS. 2006. USGS Earthquake Hazards Program. http://

earthquake.usgs.gov (accessed 20 October 2006).

63. Earthquake Kobe Japan 1995. NIST. Retrieved October 15, 2021, from https://www.nist.gov/el/earthquake-kobejapa n-1995

64. Klinenberg, E. 2002. *Heat Wave: A Social Autopsy of Disaster in Chicago.* Chicago, IL: University of Chicago Press.

65. Hemenway, D. 2005. American Females at Highest Risk for Murder. Harvard School of Public Health. https://news. harvard.edu/gazette/story/2002/04/american-females-at-highest-risk-for-murder/ (accessed 5 October 2021).

66. Bureau of Justice Statistics. 2005. Homicide Rates Recently Declined to Levels Last Seen in the Late 1960's. Department of Justice. http://www.ojp.usdoj.gov/bjs/ glance/hmrt.htm (accessed 19 July 2006).

67. U.S. Centers for Disease Control and Prevention (CDC). 2005. Sexual Violence: Fact Sheet. https://www.cdc.gov/ violenceprevention/sexualviolence/index.html (accessed 05 October 2021).

68. Department of Justice. 2004. Crime and Victim Statistics 2004. http://www.ojp.usdoj.gov/bjs/cvict.htm (accessed 19 July 2006).

69. Levitt, S. and S.J. Dubner. 2005. *Freakonomics: A Rogue Economist Explores the Hidden Side of Everything.* William Morrow/HarperCollins.

70. American Psychological Association. 2021. Violence & Youth. https://www.apa.org/pi/prevent-violence/resourc es/violence-youth.pdf (accessed 10 October 2021).

71. Monkkonen, E.H. 2001. *Murder in New York City.* Berkeley: University of California Press.

72. Calhoun, J.B. 1962. Crowding Into the Behavioral Sink. *Scientific American* 206:139-148.

73. From e-mail communication with Dr. F.B.M. De Waal on July 14, 2006.

74. Aureli, F., F.B.M. De Waal, and P.G. Judge. 2000. Coping

with Crowding. *Scientific American* 77.

75. Sampson, R.J. 2003. The neighborhood context of well-being. *Perspectives in Biology and Medicine* 46.3:53-S64.

76. Katz, L.F., J. Kling, and J.B. Liebman. 2001. Moving to Opportunity in Boston: Early Results of a Randomized Mobility Experiment. *Q. J. Econ.* 116(2):607-54.

77. Fajnzylber, P., D. Lederman, and N. Loayza. 1998. Determinants of Crime Rates in Latin America and the World. An Empirical Assessment. The World Bank. https://documents1.worldbank.org/curated/en/198251468 752978462/pdf/multi-page.pdf (accessed 05 October 2021).

78. Smith, D.M. and M.A. Zahn. 1999. *Homicide: A Sourcebook of Social Research.* London: SAGE Publications Ltd.

79. U.S. Department of Health and Human Services. (n.d.). NIMH. Suicide. National Institute of Mental Health. Retrieved October 16, 2021, from https://www.nimh.nih. gov/health/statistics/suicide

80. The Emile Durkheim Archive. 2006. Suicide. http:// durkheim.itgo.com/suicide.html (accessed 30 October 2006).

81. U.S. Department of Health and Human Services. (n.d.). NIMH. Suicide. National Institute of Mental Health. Retrieved October 16, 2021, from https://www.nimh.nih. gov/health/statistics/suicide

82. Lucy, W.H. 2003. Mortality Risk Associated with Leaving Home: Recognizing the Relevance of the Built Environment. *Am J Public Health* 93(9): 1564-1569M.

83. Media, NHTSA. (2020, December 18). NHTSA Releases 2019 Crash Fatality Data. NHTSA. Retrieved October 16, 2021, from https://www.nhtsa.gov/press-releases/nhtsareleases-2019-crash-fatality-data

84. Automobile Association of America. (n.d.). Aggressive Driving: Three Studies. http://www.aaafoundation.org/ resources/index.cfm?button=agdrtext (accessed 19 July

2006).

85. Whitlock, F.A. 1971. *Death on the Road: A Study in Social Violence.* London: Tavistock.

86. Goodman, M.F., F.D. Bents, L. Tijerina, and D. Benel. 1999. An Investigation of the Safety Implications of Wireless Communication in Vehicles. http://www.nhtsa.dot.gov/people/injury/research/wireless/ (accessed 17 July 2006).

87. Hahn, R.W., P.C. Tetlock, and J.K. Burnett. 2000. Should You Be Allowed To Use Your Cellular Phone While Driving? *Regulation* 23: 46-55.

88. Briem, V. and L.R. Hedman. 1995. Behavioural effects of mobile telephone use during simulated driving. *Ergonomics* 38: 2536-2562.

89. Strayer, D.L. et al. 2003. Cell Phone-Induced Failures of Visual Attention During Simulated Driving. *J Exp Psychol Appl.* 9(1):23-32.

90. Harbluk, J.L., Y.I. Noy, and M. Eizenman. 2002. Impact of cognitive distraction on driver visual behavior and vehicle control. Paper presented at the 81st annual meeting of the Transportation Research Board, Washington, DC.

91. Strayer, D.L. et al. 2003. Cell Phone-Induced Failures of Visual Attention During Simulated Driving.

92. McCarley, J.S., M. Vais, H. Pringle, and D.L. Strayer et al. 2001. Conversation Disrupts Visual Scanning of Traffic Scenes. Paper presented at the 9th Vision in Vehicles Conference, 2001, Brisbane, Australia.

93. National Highway Traffic Safety Administration (NHTSA). 2004. *Traffic Safety Facts 2003.* NHTSA, Washington, DC.

94. National Safety Council. 2000. *Injury Facts – 2000 Edition.* National Safety Council, Itasca, IL.

95. Pedestrian Crash Statistics. Pedestrian Safety Guide and Countermeasure Selection System. (n.d.). Retrieved October 16, 2021, from http://www.pedbikesafe.org/pedsafe/guide_statistics.cfm

96. National Highway Traffic and Safety Administration. 2004. Pedestrian Roadway Fatalities. http://www-nrd.nhtsa.dot.gov/ (accessed 19 July 2006).

97. US fire problem. NFPA. (n.d.). Retrieved October 16, 2021, from https://www.nfpa.org/News-and-Research/Data-research-and-tools/US-Fire-Problem

98. Fire loss. U.S. experience with smoke alarms and other fire detection ... (n.d.). Retrieved October 16, 2021, from https://www.researchgate.net/publication/267553848_US_Experience_with_Smoke_Alarms_and_Other_Fire_DetectionAlarm_Equipment. Fire Loss in the United States During 2020. NFPA. (n.d.). Retrieved October 16, 2021, from https://www.nfpa.org/-/media/Files/News-and-Research/Fire-statistics-and-reports/US-Fire-Problem/osFireLoss.pdf

99. Cromie, R. 1971. *The Great Chicago Fire*. Rutledge Hill Press.

100. National Fire Data Center. 2005. FEMA. http://www.usfa.fema.gov/inside-usfa/nfdc/pubs/tfrs.shtm (accessed 19 July 2006).

101. National Commission on Terrorist Attacks Upon the United States. 2006. http://www.9-11commission.gov/ (accessed 30 October 2006).

102. Wishnow, R.M. 1976. The conquest of the major infectious diseases in the United States: a bicentennial retrospect. *Annu Rev Microbiol.* 30:427-50.

103. Elflein, John. Deaths Communicable Diseases AnnuallyWorldwide 2019. Statista, 1 April 2021. https://www.statista.com/statistics/282715/deaths-fromcommunicable-diseases-worldwide/

104. Lederberg, J. 2000. Infectious History. American Association for the Advancement of Science. http://www.univie.ac.at/hygiene-aktuell/lederberg.htm (accessed 19 October 2006).

105. Institute of Medicine. 1992. Emerging Infections: Microbial

Threats to Health in the United States. https://wwwnc. cdc.gov/eid/page/20-year-timeline-infections (accessed 08 October 2021).

106. Ibid.

107. American Public Health Association. 2000. *Control of Communicable Diseases Manual.* American Public Health Association.

108. Soulsby, E. 2005. Resistance to antimicrobials in humans and animals. *Brit J Med* 331: 1219-20.

109. Maxcy, Rosenau, and Last, ed. 1998. *Public Health & Preventive Medicine.* Appleton and Lange.

110. Institute of Medicine. 1992. Emerging Infections: Microbial Threats to Health in the United States.

111. Goodell, Jeff. How Climate Change Is Ushering in a New Pandemic Era. Rolling Stone. 4 October 2021. https:// www.rollingstone.com/culture/culture-features/climate-change-risks-infectious-diseases-covid-19-eboladengue-1098923/

112. Freccero, S.P. 2005. Anthrax whodunit: Is it a cold case file? http://www.csmonitor.com/2005/1110/p09s02-coop. htm (accessed 10 October 2006).

113. Morse, S.S. 1995. Factors in the Emergence of Infectious Diseases. http://www.cdc.gov/ncidod/eid/vol1no1/morse htm#ref29(accessed 10 October 2006).

114. CDC. 2005. Trends in Tuberculosis --- United States, 1998—2003. http://www.cdc.gov/mmwr/preview/mmwrh tml/mm5310a2.htm (accessed 15 October 2006).

115. Anderson, C. 1991. Cholera epidemic traced to risk miscalculation. *Nature* 1991: 354:255.

116. Morse, S.S. 1995. Factors in the Emergence of Infectious Diseases. *EID* 1995 1:1.

117. MacKenzie, W.R., N.J. Hoxie, and M.E. Proctor et al. 1994. A Massive Outbreak in Milwaukee of Cryptosporidium Infection Transmitted through the water supply. *N Engl J*

Med 331:161-7.

118. National Academies Press. 2006. Public Health Systems and Emerging Infections: Assessing the Capabilities of the Public and Private Sectors: Workshop. http://books. nap.edu/catalog/9869.html (accessed 19 October 2006).

119. Maxcy et al. 1998. *Public Health and Preventive Medicine.*

120. CDC. (n.d.) Compendium of Measures To Prevent Disease Associated with Animals in Public Settings. http:// www.cdc.gov/mmwr/preview/mmwrhtml/rr5404a1.htm (accessed 19 October 2006).

121. American Public Health Association. 2000. *Control of Communicable Diseases Manual.* American Public Health Association.

122. CDC. 2005. Disease Vectors and Pests. http://www. cdc.gov/nceh/publications/books/housing/cha04.htm (accessed 15 October 2006).

123. Hantavirus Pulmonary Syndrome (HPS). American Lung Association. https://www.lung.org/lung-healthdiseases/ lung-disease-lookup/hantavirus-pulmonarysyndrome

124. CDC. 2006. Healthy Housing Manual. http://www.cdc. gov/nceh/publications/books/housing/2006_HHM_ FINAL_chapter_04.pdf (accessed 25 October 2006).

125. Plotts, Edwin. Pet Ownership Statistics by State, and so Much More (Updated 2020). Pawlicy Advisor. 13 November 2020. https://www.pawlicy.com/blog/us-pet-ownership-statistics/

126. *Control of Communicable Diseases Manual.*

127. Pneumococcal Pneumonia. Pneumococcal Pneumonia l American Lung Association. https://www.lung.org/lung-health-diseases/lung-disease-lookup/pneumonia/pneum ococcal

128. Influenza (Flu). American Lung Association. https:// www.lung.org/lung-health-diseases/lung-diseaselookup/ influenza

129. About Flu. Centers for Disease Control and Prevention. 15 October 2021. https://www.cdc.gov/flu/about/index. html

130. National Restaurant Association. 2005. Industry Research. http://www.restaurant.org/research/ (accessed 20 October 2006).

131. Los Angeles County Department of Health Services. 2005. Food Handler's Guide. http://lapublichealth.org/eh/ fhgde/FOODPROT.HTM (accessed 19 October 2006).

132. Mead, P.S., L. Slutsker, and V. Dietz et al. 1999. Food-Related Illness and Death in the United States. *Emerg Infect Dis.* 5(5):607-25.

133. Campylobacter (Campylobacteriosis). Centers for Disease Control and Prevention. 14 April 2021. https://www.cdc. gov/campylobacter/index.html

134. Salmonella. Centers for Disease Control and Prevention. 13 October 2021. https://www.cdc.gov/salmonella/index. html

135. E. Coli (Escherichia Coli). Centers for Disease Control and Prevention. 15 September 2021. https://www.cdc.gov/ ecoli/index.html

136. Hepatitis A. Centers for Disease Control and Prevention. 22 June 2020. https:// www.cdc.gov/hepatitis/hav/index. htm

137. CDC. 2006. Toxoplasmosis Fact Sheet. http://www. cdc.gov/ncidod/dpd/parasites/toxoplasmosis/factsht_ toxoplasmosis.htm (accessed 20 October 2006).

138. CDC. 2021. Listeria (Listeriosis). https://www.cdc.gov/list eria/index.html?CDC_AA_refVal=https%3A%2F%2Fww w.cdc.gov%2Fpulsenet%2Fpathogens%2Flisteria.html (accessed 10 October 2021).

139. Craun, G.F., N. Nwachuku, R.L. Calderon, and M.F. Craun. 2002. Outbreaks in drinking-water systems, 1991-1998. *Journal of Environmental Health* 65:16-25.

140. Surveillance Overview | Statistics Center | HIV/AIDS | CDC. https://www.cdc.gov/hiv/statistics/surveillance/index.html
141. Heitz, D. 2020, April 24. HIV by the Numbers: Facts, Statistics, and You. Retrieved January 06, 2020.
142. Understanding HIV. National Institutes of Health. U.S. Department of Health and Human Services. https://hivinfo.nih.gov/understanding-hiv
143. Sexually Transmitted Diseases (STDs). Centers for Disease Control and Prevention. 17 June 2021. https://www.cdc.gov/std/default.htm
144. CDC. 2006. Avian Influenza. http://www.cdc.gov/flu/avian/ (accessed 20 October 2006).
145. CDC. 2006. SARS. http://www.cdc.gov/ncidod/sars/ (accessed 25 October 2006).
146. SARS could come back. Armenian Medical Network. http://www.health.am/2003e/01/177.php
147. CDC. 2005. West Nile Virus. http://www.cdc.gov/ncidod/dvbid/westnile/index.htm (accessed 25 October 2006).
148. Tuberculosis (TB). Centers for Disease Control and Prevention. 4 May 2016. https://www.cdc.gov/tb/publications/factsheets/drtb/mdrtb.htm
149. Tuberculosis. World Health Organization. https://www.who.int/news-room/fact-sheets/detail/tuberculosis
150. Williams, N. 1997. New studies affirm BSE-human link. *Science.* 278: 31.
151. Bovine Spongiform Encephalopathy (BSE). Centers for Disease Control and Prevention. 10 September 2021. https://www.cdc.gov/prions/bse/index.html
152. Viral Hemorrhagic Fevers (VHFs). Centers for Disease Control and Prevention. 2 September 2021. https://www.cdc.gov/vhf/index.html
153. Newport, B.F. 2020, November 23. Americans Big on Idea of Living in the Country. Gallup.

154. Ingraham, C., *The Washington Post*. 2018. The Size of The Town You Live in Has a Huge Effect on Happiness Levels. ScienceAlert. https://www.sciencealert.com/where-you-live-has-a-drastic-effect-on-your-happiness-levels (accessed 10 October 2021).

155. Schaefer, Annette. 2005. Commuting Takes Its Toll. *Scientific American*, 1 October. www.scientificamerican.com/article/commuting-takes-its-toll

156. About Social Determinants of Health (SDOH). 2020, August 19. Retrieved January 28, 2021, from https://www.cdc.gov/socialdeterminants/about.html

157. Sawhill, Isabel V. Social Capital: Why We Need It and How We Can Create More of It. Brookings, 22 July 2020. https://www.brookings.edu/research/socialcapital-why-we-need-it-and-how-we-can-create-more-of-it/

158. https://www.jec.senate.gov/public/index.cfm/republicans/2018/4/the-geography-of-social-capital-in-america

159. Seymour, Valentine. The Human-Nature Relationship and Its Impact on Health: A Critical Review. Frontiers in Public Health, Frontiers Media S.A. 18 November 2016. https://www.ncbi.nlm.nih.gov/pmc/articles/PMC5114301/

160. How The Dust Bowl Made Americans Refugees in Their Own Country. 2019. [online] Available at: https://www.history.com/news/dust-bowl-migrants-california (accessed 09 January 2021).

161. McCann, A. 2020, March 09. Happiest Cities in America. Retrieved February 02, 2021, from https://wallethub.com/edu/happiest-places-to-live/32619

162. Wallace, N. 2016, November 29. The Best Ski Towns in America – 2015 Edition. Retrieved January 30, 2021, from https://smartasset.com/mortgage/americas-best-ski-towns

163. Methodology. 2020. Retrieved February 07, 2021, from https://livability.com/best-places/top-100-best-places-to-live/2020/methodology

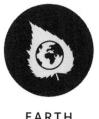

**EARTH
BOOKS**

ENVIRONMENT

Earth Books are practical, scientific and philosophical publications about our relationship with the environment. Earth Books explore sustainable ways of living; including green parenting, gardening, cooking and natural building. They also look at ecology, conservation and aspects of environmental science, including green energy. An understanding of the interdependence of all living things is central to Earth Books, and therefore consideration of our relationship with other animals is important. Animal welfare is explored. The purpose of Earth Books is to deepen our understanding of the environment and our role within it. The books featured under this imprint will both present thought-provoking questions and offer practical solutions.

If you have enjoyed this book, why not tell other readers by posting a review on your preferred book site.

Recent bestsellers from Earth Books are:

In Defence of Life
Essays on a Radical Reworking of Green Wisdom
Julian Rose
Julian Rose's book has the power to lift the reader into another dimension. He offers a way to break through the destructive patterns of our consumer-obsessed society and discover a simpler, more fulfilling way forward.
Paperback: 978-1-78279-257-4 ebook: 978-1-78279-256-7

Eyes of the Wild
Journeys of Transformation with the Animal Powers
Eleanor O'Hanlon
The ancient understanding of animals as guides to self knowledge and the soul comes alive through close encounters with some of the most magnificent creatures of the wild.
Paperback: 978-1-84694-957-9 ebook: 978-1-84694-958-6

Simplicity Made Easy
Jennifer Kavanagh
Stop wishing your life was more simple, and start making it happen! With the help of Jennifer Kavanagh's book, turn your focus to what really matters in life.
Paperback: 978-1-84694-543-4 ebook: 978-1-84694-895-4

Acorns Among the Grass
Adventures in Eco-Therapy
Caroline Brazier
When we reconnect with the natural world, we discover our deep relationship with life. This book embraces the ways in which environmental work nourishes us, psychologically and spiritually.
Paperback: 978-1-84694-619-6 ebook: 978-1-84694-883-1

Safe Planet
Renewable Energy Plus Workers' Power
John Cowsill
Safe Planet lays out a roadmap of renewable energy sources
and meteorological data to direct us towards a safe planet.
Paperback: 978-1-78099-682-0 ebook: 978-1-78099-683-7

GreenSpirit
Path to a New Consciousness
Marian Van Eyk McCain
A collection of essays on 21st Century green spirituality and its
key role in creating a peaceful and sustainable world.
Paperback: 978-1-84694-290-7 ebook: 978-1-78099-186-3

This Is Hope
Green Vegans and the New Human Ecology
How We Find Our Way to a Humane and Environmentally
Sane Future.
Will Anderson
This Is Hope compares the outcomes of two human ecologies;
one is tragic, the other full of promise...
Paperback: 978-1-78099-890-9

Readers of ebooks can buy or view any of these bestsellers by
clicking on the live link in the title. Most titles are published
in paperback and as an ebook. Paperbacks are available in
traditional bookshops. Both print and ebook formats are
available online.

Find more titles and sign up to our readers' newsletter at
http://www.johnhuntpublishing.com/non-fiction
Follow us on Facebook at
https://www.facebook.com/JHPNonFiction